P9-AGW-711

i

HEARING LOSS
Facts and Fiction

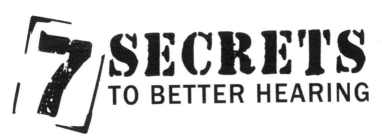

HEARING LOSS
[FACTS] and FICTION
7 SECRETS TO BETTER HEARING

Timothy Frantz, M.D.

I dedicate this book to over 40 million people in the United States who suffer from hearing loss (possibly without even knowing it).

This book is also dedicated to Dr. Raymond L. Hilsinger, Jr., Dr. Barry Rasgon, Dr. Raul Cruz, and Dr. Frederick Byl. They are the ENT professors who believed in me and imparted their knowledge, skills, and passion for treatment of patients with ear disease and hearing loss.

DISCLAIMER This publication is intended to provide educational, helpful, and informative material. It is not intended to diagnose, treat, cure, or prevent any health problems or hearing loss condition, nor is it intended to replace the advice of a licensed hearing professional. No action should be taken solely on the contents of this book. Always consult a qualified health-care professional on any matters regarding your hearing and before adopting any suggestions or drawing inferences from the content of this book. The author and publisher specifically disclaim all responsibility for any liability, loss or risk, personal or otherwise, which is incurred as a consequence, directly or indirectly, from the use, adoption or application of any contents of this book without the recommendation of a qualified professional. Any and all product names referenced within this book are the trademarks of their respective owners. None of these owners have sponsored, authorized, endorsed, or approved this book. Always read all information provided by the manufacturer before using any device or product. The author and publisher are not responsible for claims made by manufacturers. The statements made in this book have not been evaluated by the United States Food and Drug Administration, and are solely based on over 20 years of Dr. Frantz's experience working as an otolaryngologist and a hearing aid dispenser in the hearing profession.

Copyright © 2014 by Timothy Frantz

All rights reserved. In accordance with the U.S. copyright Act of 1976, the scanning, uploading, and electronic sharing of any part of this book without the permission of the publisher constitute unlawful piracy and theft of the author's intellectual property. If you would like to use material from the book (other than for review purposes), prior written permission must be obtained by contacting the publisher at info@theheardoc.com. Thank you for your support of the author's rights.

THD Publishing | P.O. Box 338 Red Bluff, California 96080
Printed in the United States of America

Second Edition: September 2014 Library of Congress Cataloging-in-Publication Data- Frantz, Timothy Hearing Loss: facts and fiction / Timothy Frantz –2nd ed., 228pp. Includes bibliographical references and index.

ISBN **978-0-9908543-0-2**

1. Hearing loss. 2. Hearing loss treatment. 3. Communication. 4. Hearing aids

ACKNOWLEDGEMENTS

I would like to express my gratitude to my patients who encouraged me to write this book.

Above all I want to thank my wife, Kimberli, and my children. They supported and encouraged me in spite of all the time writing this book took me away from them.

I would also like to thank my trusted friend, Stephen Fry, and his team at Spindustry Digital which includes Tom Ambroson and Howard Tempero. I appreciate their expertise and professionalism in the process of design and writing of this book.

I am also forever grateful to Edward L. Applebaum, M.D. who graciously allowed me to observe him in the operating suite as a wide-eyed third year medical student, and showed me for the first time the miracle of hearing restoration surgery.

Last, but not least, I want to thank Dr. William Nicol and his wife, Anne, for their encouragement and editorial assistance; and the GN Resound Corporation for permission to use their images.

TABLE OF CONTENTS

....

"Whoever has ears to hear, let them hear…"

-Jesus Christ

....

PREFACE

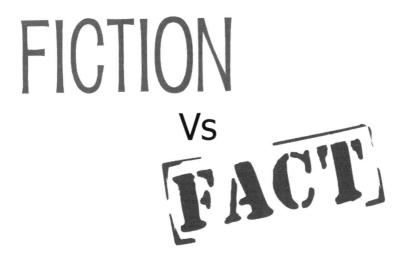

Throughout this book you will read "Fact" and "Fiction" statements. These are intended to help you stop and think about the different subjects and topics covered in the book. Read the fiction statements and if they sound like you, take a moment and think about taking the next step which is to set up an appointment with a local hearing professional. If you need advice, guidance or recommendations – feel free to call, email me at **info@theheardoc.com** or subscribe to my free newsletter available at **www.theheardoc.com**.

If you want to hear better, you have already taken the first step by buying this book.

Here, I give you the tools you need to help identify if you have hearing loss and help you understand how to improve your hearing.

You will:
- **Learn about hearing loss**
- **Recognize if you have hearing loss**
- **Understand how to hear better**
- **Communicate more effectively**
- **Learn how to navigate the often confusing hearing aid industry**
- **Discover the 7 secrets to better hearing**

You will also become familiar with what a hearing test consists of and, if you have already had a hearing test, I will show you how to interpret your results. In addition, you will learn about the different types of hearing loss and be more informed about what can be done to correct the loss. I will also teach you some easy "active listening strategies" that will help you communicate more effectively and meaningfully with or without the use of hearing aids.

According to a recent study, nearly one in five Americans over the age of 12 years has hearing loss. The number of individuals who have hearing loss in at least one ear is estimated at 48 million. This number is steadily increasing year over year as the "baby boomers" (those born between the years 1943 and 1963) age. Fifty-five million people in the U.S. are over 55 years of age and 34 million are over 65 years old - and that figure will double by 2030. It is well known that the incidence of hearing loss increases with advancing age. In addition, many baby boomers have grown up in the era of rock concerts, nightclubs, sporting events and increasing industrial noise, all of which can damage hearing.

I have been practicing medicine as an Ear, Nose and Throat physician (otolaryngologist) commonly known as an "ENT physician," since 1991. In addition, I have also been a licensed hearing aid dispenser for over twenty years. I have literally helped thousands of patients hear better in my practice by providing medical and surgical treatments, and with hearing aids. Unfortunately, up to 75% of individuals with hearing loss do not treat it, primarily due to the high cost of hearing aids. I am genuinely concerned about what I consider to be a true crisis. In this book, I give you the tools you need to identify if you have a hearing loss, understand how to improve your hearing, know how to navigate the often confusing hearing aid industry, and learn how to communicate more effectively. Untreated hearing loss can result in relationship stress, decreased earnings, social isolation, dementia and even depression. I outline the steps to better hearing with easy-to-understand medical information, encouragement, and personal anecdotes. Based on my experience as an ENT physician, I give you the information you need to experience life fully and improve your overall quality of life by simply treating your hearing loss.

I wrote this book for several reasons. First, I wanted to help as many people as possible hear better and I realized that much of the information I share on a daily basis with my patients during one-on-one medical consultations could be easily written in a book. Second, I wanted to dispel many of the myths and falsehoods about hearing loss and hearing aids which I often hear from patients and their families, hence the subtitle, "Facts and Fiction." This book is especially written for the person who thinks that he or she may have hearing loss but is hesitant to take the next step and seek help. I also wrote to those who are in denial of their hearing loss, since hearing loss usually occurs gradually over time and patients generally learn to compensate for the hearing loss in different ways. Along with the fact-and-fiction statements which you will find in this book, there are dozens of secrets to better hearing in each section. I discuss many of these with my patients during consultations each day and now I share them with you. I strongly believe that knowledge of the importance of hearing and the functions of the ear is an essential starting place.

You will also learn the process of selecting and purchasing hearing aids (without spending your entire life savings). The hearing aid industry can be complicated and confusing. There are hundreds of different styles, functions, prices, and settings for hearing aids. My patients are inundated with full page newspaper and direct mail ads for "fully digital hearing aids," "invisible hearing aids," and "feature-rich hearing aids." I feel that many of these ads create further confusion. In this book I help you navigate through this confusing hearing aid information, explain how the hearing aid industry operates and let you in on some secrets to buying hearing aids that will save you money and get you hearing clearly again.

You may have normal hearing and picked up this book looking for answers to help you cope with a family member, spouse or friend with hearing loss. Conversations and relationships can be quite frustrating when one person suffers from hearing loss. The person with hearing loss may not even realize just how bad it is. Many learn to cope with their hearing loss by replying to questions with stock phrases such as, "uh-huh" or "yes honey" or even worse won't respond at all. Many may be too proud to ask you to repeat. This book is written for you too.

I have included helpful information about hearing loss that will enable you to help your family member or friend get the help he/she needs. I also have suggestions for you to maximize your communication with someone who has hearing loss (see "Active Listening Measures" appendix in back of book.)

Finally, in this book I will tell you the seven secrets (and dozens more) to better hearing that everyone should know. Everyone can hear better by using these 7 simple secrets to better hearing.

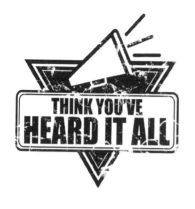

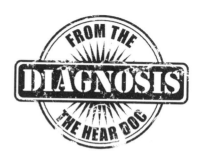

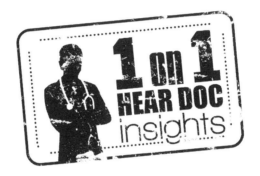

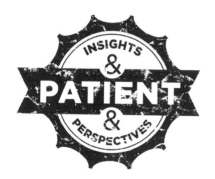

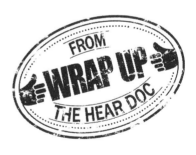

Keep a look out for these callouts throughout the book to get unique perspectives and insights that keep you turning pages.

Taking the conversational approach. . .

Nobody likes to be lectured to, especially when it comes to medical-related content. Ok, well maybe I like to go to lectures on this subject, but that is rooted in my passion for my profession. You will notice a series of callouts throughout this book, which are labeled as follows:

- **Diagnosis From The Hear Doc**
- **Think You've Heard it All**
- **One-On-One Hear Doc Insights**
- **Patient Insights & Perspectives**
- **Wrap Up from The Hear Doc**

These callouts are used to call your attention to specific informational tidbits that I want to especially mention in this book. This will also keep this book from becoming a medical dissertation and allow for more informational engagement. In some instances, these callouts allow for an anecdotal story that you may be able to relate to (or laugh at). This book is designed to educate you via a conversation with you about hearing loss. My goal is to have you close this book and feel like you have had a private consultation with me. Hopefully, I will answer all your questions and dispel myths about hearing loss. Then, I want you to take the next step and schedule an appointment with a hearing professional in your area to get the help you need.

Now sit down...and tell me...how can I help you today?

"I may have hearing loss, but it does not affect my day-to-day activities or relationships."

FICTION

Even if you think you have a hearing loss, you are probably already missing out on much of life.

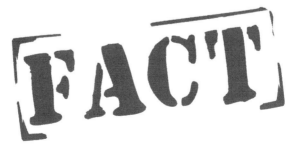

SECTION 1

The Basics - From Ear to Hear

This section contains everything you need to know about communication, hearing, and the inner workings and complexities of the ear. There will also be information covered that you may not need to know, but I am passionate about the subject of hearing and have been known to get carried away at times.

The following topics will be covered in this section:

- The Importance of Hearing
- Recognizing if You have Hearing Loss
- Understanding How We Hear
- Steps to Take for Hearing Loss Prevention
- Earwax is Important (it is not dirt!)

Hearing problems are mainly in
the elderly population.

FICTION

There are currently over 48 million
people in the U.S. who suffer from
hearing loss and the majority (over 65%)
are less than 65 years of age.

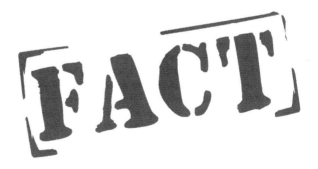

CHAPTER 1

The Importance of Hearing

I believe that no method of communication is as meaningful and effective as hearing another's voice. However, we all know there are many ways to communicate with people in addition to audibly hearing others and listening. These include:

- Written communication (like this book)
- Written letters/notes
- Email
- Sign Language (ASL)
- Texting
- Telecommunication Devices for the Deaf (TDD)
- Body language
- Touching
- Lip reading

Starting when you are still in your mother's womb, hearing develops and communication starts. As we grow, it becomes of absolute importance throughout our lifetime in all of our relationships. Most doctors agree that by 25 weeks gestation, when you weighed only about a pound, you were able to hear your mother's/father's voices and recognize them. Research has shown that an unborn baby's heart rate often slows when its mother is speaking, a sign that the baby not only hears, but recognizes the sound and is calmed by it. Unborn babies also often move in response to certain sounds, particularly loud sounds.

In the U.S. nearly all children are tested for hearing loss at birth. If a hearing loss is found, babies as young as 2-3 months can begin wearing hearing aids that subsequently support the development of normal speech and allow them to excel in school. Children learn to speak by listening to those around them and by imitating vocal intonations and speech patterns of their parents and others in their environment. The earliest words spoken by most infants are "Dada" or "Mama."

Older children and young adults also need to hear their mothers' voice. According to Sarah H. Lee in a recent Huffington Post article, "In 2010 researchers found that young girls who talked to their mothers, either on the phone or face-to-face, experienced a drop in the stress hormone cortisol. Their brains also released a burst of oxytocin, the neuromodulator responsible for feelings of love and pleasure. The results of the study led one of its architects, Leslie Seltzer, a psychologist at the University of Wisconsin, to wonder about the precise origins of Mom's power to soothe. Was it a maternal ability to say the right thing? Or did it have to do with the tempo, pitch, tone, stress, and rhythm of her voice – some quasi-musical property of mom talk that runs parallel to common sense."

"http://www.huffingtonpost.com/2012/01/11/sound-of-moms-voice_n_1200003.html

Hearing is also essential for developing all meaningful relationships. "Hearing empowers us and enriches our lives. Hearing enables us to socialize, work, interact, communicate, and even relax. Good hearing also helps to keep us safe, warning us of potential danger or alerting us to someone else's distress. Hearing is essential for us to be able to live and participate in life more fully. Problems with our hearing may lead to feelings of isolation and even depression. Our hearing provides us with an enormous source of information, some of it obvious and some we barely notice, but when combined, this information forms the bridge between the world and how we interact with it."

http://www.oticon.com/hearing/facts/hearing/why-is-hearing-important.aspx

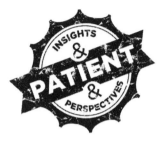

As a child I lived in a small town in rural Illinois, and my grandmother, "Omi", and aunt lived with us at the time. Omi had been completely blind for two and a half decades due to an eye condition. Despite her handicap, she adapted well and had a full life. She had many friends and acquaintances with whom she would socialize. My grandmother had a keen sense of hearing, upon which she completely relied to interact with her environment and with others. Omi loved talking on the telephone. In fact, she would spend hours and hours each day talking to friends and other family members. She also "read" many books, which were actually books on cassette tape (considered audiobooks today) or she read braille books with her fingers. My grandmother and I had a great relationship; she would always listen to me tell her about my experiences in school and she would often give me advice on life. My Omi is long gone now, but I still treasure the conversations about life that I was able to have with her. Her hearing compensated for her loss of vision.

"Blindness separates us from things, but Deafness separates us from people." – Helen Keller

Hearing is essential in business relationships.

A recent study by Sergei Kochkin, Ph.D., in May 2007 of the Better Hearing Institute, Washington D.C. called, "The Impact of Untreated Hearing Loss on Household Income" showed:

"In a survey of more than 40,000 households utilizing the Family Opinion panel, hearing loss was shown to negatively impact household income on-average up to $12,000 per year depending on the degree of hearing loss. However, the use of hearing instruments was shown to mitigate the [financial] effects of hearing loss by 50%. For America's 24 million hearing-impaired adults who do not use hearing instruments, the impact of untreated hearing loss is quantified to be in excess of $100 billion annually. At a 15% tax bracket, the cost to society could be well in excess of $18 billion due to unrealized taxes."

Hearing is essential for you to have a successful marriage.

Fifteen years ago, my wife and I were in a rough spot in our marriage. We met with a marriage counselor weekly for about 18 months. The most important thing we learned during that time was how to communicate with one another. My wife and I are both busy physicians and, at that time in our marriage, we were not communicating in a meaningful way on a daily basis. The counselor challenged us to have an uninterrupted 15 minute time each day to simply verbally communicate to each other how we felt about our lives that day (i.e. I feel [Fill in the blank] today ... sad, thrilled, sexy, angry, neglected, etc.). We were encouraged to really hear and listen to each other. It worked. We just celebrated our twenty-seventh wedding anniversary! Today, we have a vibrant marriage and regularly hear (and listen to) each other's concerns and feelings with empathy. It has become an important part of our daily lives and I truly believe it saved our marriage and sustains it to this day.

All relationships have their ups and downs, but I believe that through effective communication, you can resolve most issues; or, at least, agree to disagree. In my opinion, when it comes to a marriage, it's not just communication that helps, but effective, truthful, honest sharing of feelings which are communicated, even if for only a few minutes each day.

"We have two ears and one mouth so that we can listen twice as much as we speak." – Epictetus

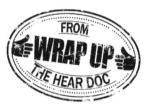

Our hearing is a precious sense. Certainly, good hearing allows us to communicate with others in our lives, but it is also critical for socialization, recreation, overall health, work, and for safety. Now that you, hopefully, understand the importance and impact of having good hearing, let's take the next step and look at hearing loss and then determine if you have any symptoms of it.

"My hearing is just fine. I always know when someone is speaking to me, but I don't always understand what is being said, especially when I'm in a noisy room."

FICTION

When family and friends complain that the TV volume is too loud, this is often one of the most common first signs of hearing loss. When you set the volume at a comfortable level for yourself, you have no idea how it sounds to others with normal hearing.

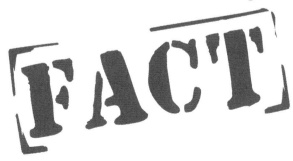

CHAPTER 2

Do You Have Hearing Loss?

Do you have hearing loss? Do you seem to be able to hear when someone is speaking but are not able to understand what is being said? The most common phrases I hear as a physician from patients with hearing loss are:

"She always mumbles..."

"He never listens to me..."

"My wife speaks too quietly..."

"I can hear him, but I can't understand..."

"I hear just fine, unless I'm in a noisy room..."

"He turns up the TV volume too loud..."

"He always talks too loud..."

Have you heard or said any of these phrases and are you 55 years of age or older? Then you probably have some form of hearing loss, and if you do, you're not alone. In the United States there are over 48 million Americans with hearing loss in at least one ear.

If you have experienced any of the following scenarios, your chance of hearing loss is even greater:

- Prolonged exposure to loud noise during any period of life

- A history of chronic ear infections

- A family history of hearing loss

- A history of chemotherapy or ototoxic drugs

- Previous head injury

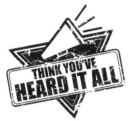

Here are some interesting statistics - hearing loss is the third most common health condition affecting older adults, after hypertension and arthritis. Hearing loss is usually slow to develop, although occasionally it occurs suddenly. Usually, hearing loss gradually progresses over a period of many years. Most patients first notice hearing problems 7-8 years before they finally seek help for their hearing loss.

In my hearing clinic, we have a "Hearing Ability Assessment Questionnaire" that is completed by every patient with possible hearing loss. This form asks some simple questions which help me to determine whether or not a patient has hearing loss. There are ten questions on the questionnaire and I determine the likelihood of a hearing loss based on the number of positive responses.

Take a moment now and answer these same questions. . .

Hearing Ability
Assessment Questionnaire

This questionnaire asks some simple questions which help me to determine whether or not a patient has hearing loss. These ten questions help me determine the likelihood of hearing loss based on the number of positive responses:

Do you have difficulty understanding speech in a group?

Do you hear people speaking but not understand them?

Do you ask people to repeat themselves?

Do others raise their voices to help you hear them?

Do you have to turn the TV up louder than normal?

Do you concentrate so much to listen that you tire from it?

Do you ever avoid situations because of your hearing?

Do you have difficulty understanding conversations in the car?

Do you have difficulty understanding on the phone?

Do you hear some people's voices better than others?

If you answered "Yes" to two or more of these questions, there is a high likelihood that you suffer from hearing loss. Probably the question that is answered "Yes" most often is: "Do you have difficulty understanding speech in a group?" The second most common positive response I hear is: "Do you hear people speaking but not understand them?"

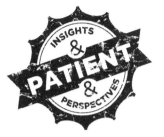

In my practice, I have seen patients with severe to profound loss of hearing in both ears on the hearing test, surprisingly, mark only one or two (out of ten) positive responses on the hearing questionnaire. Clearly they are in denial of their hearing loss and are very resistant to letting me help them with surgery or hearing aids. In contrast, patients who mark eight to ten positive responses on the questionnaire are generally accepting of their hearing loss and are eager to do something about it. Which category of patient are you? Do you freely admit you have a hearing problem and desire to hear better, or are you in denial of a hearing loss?

Often the patients I see with hearing loss are brought in by a spouse or a family member who is insisting that I "do something" about the patient's hearing. The person who is in denial of his/her hearing loss is one of the most difficult situations for me to deal with in my medical practice. I start by sitting down and explaining the hearing test results with the patient, to make sure they truly understand the test results. Usually the hearing loss has developed over many years and the individual has adapted to the hearing loss. When he/she does not hear someone clearly, he/she generally will ignore the speaker, or adopts the practice of simply replying "Yes" or "Uh - huh," rather than ask the speaker to repeat. These patients are usually excellent lip readers, without ever having taken formal training. If you are that type of patient, I am here to tell you I am glad that you found this book and that you are in good hands. I will also tell you that if you answered "Yes" to two or more questions in the previous questionnaire, you probably have a hearing disability (whether you want to hear that or not) and I can help you.

The most common type of hearing loss in over 95% of my adult patients is called sensorineural hearing loss (or "nerve deafness"). In this condition, there are usually no surgical procedures which I can perform or medications I can prescribe to help restore hearing, except in the case of profound deafness in both ears in which case cochlear implants can be considered (see chapter 9 - more later). Usually, the physical examination of the ears and ear structures is completely normal.

In the vast majority of my adult patients with hearing loss, hearing aids are required. Most patients are receptive to considering hearing aids, but not everyone. Patients who are in denial of their hearing loss generally are hoping that I will find a large ball of wax in their ears (which has been present for years) and after removal they will hear normally again. Unfortunately, this is almost never the case. I discuss the option of using hearing aids to patients in denial of their hearing loss, and they are often very resistant to wearing them. Usually they tell me that their "wife mumbles" or "speaks too softly". They blame others for their inability to hear clearly, rather than get the help they really need for themselves. One of the most important jobs I have as an ear doctor is to (gently) convince this type of person that the problem is *their* hearing loss and that they need to accept it before I can help them. I have found in my practice, that if patients in denial regarding hearing loss leave my office without getting the help they need (usually hearing aids), they will not see me again for another consultation for 18 months! This means that these patients are living their lives with a hearing disability unnecessarily for a year and a half. Who knows how many countless moments in their daily lives will be missed or will not be as fulfilling because of lack of hearing ability, and therefore, lack of interpersonal communication.

If this type of patient brings a spouse or a friend along, I usually tell the spouse that the patient is not ignoring them and that they have a hearing disability, and not unlike other disabilities, the spouse must make some accommodations to help them communicate effectively. I frequently use the example of a person who has mobility issues. If a mobility impaired patient needs a wheelchair to get from point A to point B, surely their spouse would be accommodating and help push them around. The spouse would never say, "get out of your wheelchair and walk over here yourself!" No….they would probably assist them in an understanding way. A hearing disability is no different.

There are many things a spouse can do to help enable effective conversation. None of these things will cost you a nickel. These are simple measures to facilitate communication and are called "active listening measures." These ten tips will help any person with hearing loss hear others better and facilitate effective communication without even using hearing aids.

Active Listening Measures

1. Turn off the TV/radio if you need to have an important conversation.

2. Move to the same room if possible. Do not try to have conversations between floors of your home or from one room to the next. Have conversations in places where you can be close to the other person(s).

3. Move to a quiet room with the least amount of background noise.

4. Tell others that you have a hearing loss.

5. Try to face others who are speaking (ideally 3 to 4 feet apart). I often hear stories of a spouse who "will not listen" even though one spouse is watching TV in the family room and the other is in the kitchen 30 feet away noisily preparing food!

6. Watch each other's faces/lips. Make sure there is adequate lighting to do this. Visual cues are very important to a person with hearing loss and can help you understand what is being said. Take advantage of the lip reading skills that you may have naturally learned over the years without even knowing it!

7. If you do not understand something that is said, ask for it to be repeated.

8. Have important conversations when you are well-rested and attentive.

9. Ask for important information in writing.

10. If you have hearing aids, wear them! Studies show that almost half of hearing aids are not worn on a daily basis.

These 10 tips will help any two people hear each other better and facilitate effective communication even without medical treatment or the use of hearing aids.

There are many reasons why people do not receive the hearing health care they need and why many do not wear hearing aids when needed. But take this most important advice from a physician that specializes in hearing: *if you have hearing aids, wear them and if you need hearing aids, get them!*

Unfortunately, there still exists a stigma with wearing hearing aids. Many people recall their "granddad's hearing aids"… huge beige, banana-shaped devices situated behind granddad's ears with large brown-stained tubing connected to ugly, ear-filling, earwax stained, molded plastic inserts. Or they remember the screeching feedback that could be heard from an adjacent room! The assumption is that hearing aids will make an individual look "old". This is simply no longer the case. Hearing aids are attractive, invisible (or almost invisible), and yet are quite powerful today, allowing all ages to be active.

Many people are simply too proud to wear hearing aids. They consider those who wear them to be weak, when actually the opposite is true. A strong person communicates effectively with others, and enriches his/her life and the lives of those around them. Wearing hearing aids increases an individual's sense of control over life's events.

Look at the picture at the top of the page to your right. Now ask yourself - What do all the images have in common (* hint you won't be able to see it).

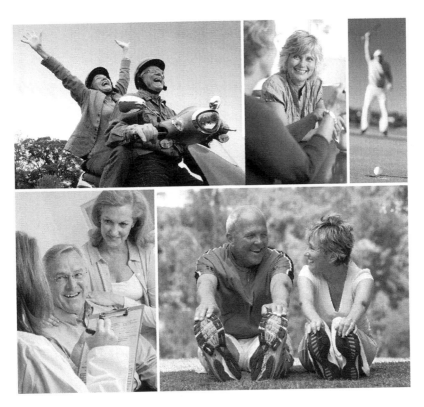

Believe it or not, people of all ages—doing all these different activities and enjoying life—can and do wear hearing aids!

Many people are in denial of their hearing loss. Between you and me, the initial acceptance is the biggest hurdle to hearing better… admitting that you have a problem. I have often noticed that many of the same people who are in denial of their hearing loss and will not wear hearing aids are the same people who are willing to accept vision loss and do wear glasses!

As mentioned previously, many people with long-term hearing loss can actually read lips fairly well, despite the lack of any formal training. While using lip reading, body language, and some verbal cues, they can usually "get by" without a hearing aid to improve their hearing. This usually takes a very understanding spouse and friends, but also can create much frustration.

Some people with hearing loss will not even consider an evaluation of their hearing due to the assumption that hearing aids are too costly. This is not true. There are hearing aids available to fit every budget. There are also many financing programs available through organizations such as CareCredit® that offer zero percent financing for the first 6 months. Of course, there are technologically superior hearing aids loaded with features such as Bluetooth®, remote control, streaming TV, dual microphones, and other expensive features which can cost thousands of dollars. A good hearing aid which will fit most hearing losses need not cost more than $800. The average lifespan of a new digital hearing aid is 6.6 years. That breaks down to only about 33 cents per ear per day. That's much cheaper than your daily cup of coffee from the local café!

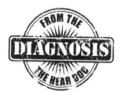

When talking about the lack of interest in hearing evaluation with some patients, I have found that there are a series of perceived mechanical problems with hearing aids, such as: feedback noise, need to replace batteries, and earwax buildup problems. These are problems of the past (and are now all urban legends that are no longer barriers). Advanced feedback suppression, digital programming, earwax traps, and in-the-ear receivers have virtually eliminated these common misperceptions.

Hearing aid batteries have also advanced. The average battery life for a hearing aid worn daily is now 6-9 days and that is improving all the time. Current battery design with Zinc/Air provides a long insertion tab attached to the battery that can be used to easily insert the battery into the aid. Several hearing aid manufacturers have also designed rechargeable hearing aids which do not require replacement of batteries for several months! And now, almost all hearing aids have simple but elegantly designed "wax traps," that are easily removed and replaced to eliminate earwax issues for the majority of hearing aid wearers.

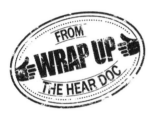

Please don't be the person who denies existing hearing loss. Unfortunately, you may not even truly know how much a hearing loss is really affecting your life and just how much you are missing in your everyday interactions with others. Swallow your pride, get a hearing test, and try a pair of hearing aids. You'll be glad you did! Today's hearing aids are discrete, high-tech devices that are affordable, easy to use and last for many years, if cared for properly. Hearing aids enrich your life, increase your earnings, increase your self-confidence and are easy to care for.

If you are a spouse, family member or friend looking out for the care of another with hearing loss, take time to have a meaningful discussion with him/her about the problem. Don't nag them about hearing loss. Discuss specific circumstances. Ask them: "Do you remember the time when you couldn't understand me in the restaurant?" Allow them to come to their own conclusions on hearing loss.

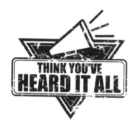

There is an interesting trend I have noticed through my own practice regarding hearing loss. In the female patients I see who live to over 90 years of age, they seem to have relatively good hearing abilities. This trait appears to be genetically passed down to other family members who frequently also have excellent hearing abilities late into life. I believe that the gene for life longevity is somehow linked to the gene for well-preserved hearing. I have always thought that it would be an interesting scientific study to perform. Unfortunately, I have not had the time to do this study yet, but perhaps in the future I will. If you are interested in participating, please feel free to email me, and maybe if I get enough of a test pool, that will be my next project

....

"The art of conversation is the art of hearing as well
as of being heard."

-William Hazlitt

....

"Everyone tends to mumble and not speak clearly, but my hearing is fine."

FICTION

The most common pattern of hearing loss which is due to aging is called presbycusis. In this condition, the hearing loss is usually in the higher tones, with the lower tones preserved. The higher sounds are critical for speech understanding. A person with this type of hearing loss will usually be able to hear speech, but not always understand what is being said.

FACT

Chapter 3
How Do We Hear?

Basics of Your Hearing Mechanism – Anatomy/Physiology 101

The hearing sense is a simple, yet incredibly complex mechanism. As a physician, I have studied it for decades and I still do not fully understand how our ears hear sounds and translate those sounds into complex language, songs, and intonation, not to mention how our brains can remember certain voices, sounds, and songs for our entire lives. Regardless of these amazing physiologic feats, here's a brief course on the human ear that I call, Ear Anatomy/Physiology 101. A warning to you, some of this description gets pretty technical. If you can, stick with me because this information will help you better understand what's going on in your ears.

It all starts with a sound….

Sound contains energy. It travels in waves with alternate compression (squeezing) of air molecules one after another. How close one sound wave is to the next sound wave determines its wavelength or frequency. Sound can travel through many different substances other than air, such as liquids like water, and solids like metal (think of train rails). Sound contains energy when it is produced. Do you remember the Memorex TV commercial with Ella Fitzgerald's voice shattering a fine wine glass? Her voice produced energy at a specific frequency which was concentrated by the wineglass, causing vibrations in the glass which, in turn, lead to the glass breaking. Sounds are produced with your voice box (larynx), palate, tongue, teeth and lips. The sound waves produced by talking and singing travel through the air at different frequencies. Humans can hear sounds as low as 20 cycles per second (20 Hertz) to as high as 20,000 cycles per second (20,000 Hertz). Animals hear slightly different frequencies than humans, for instance, a dog can hear up to 30,000 Hertz.

When a sound wave enters your ear it is first concentrated by your outer ear, also called the pinna or auricle. The outer ear is the visible portion of your ear (you might use it to hang earrings or rest your eyeglasses on). When I examine a patient who is wearing earrings, the patient often asks if she should take them out for the examination. My answer is usually that this is not necessary. These days, the hearing tools I use are quite sophisticated. Just imagine what the gemstones in your earrings look like under my high-powered operating microscope, sparkling under the bright light source!

The human outer ear has a unique shape that is specific to the characteristics of the human voice. It actually preferentially collects the speech frequencies best between 2,000 – 6,000 Hz, which are essential in speech comprehension. The sounds which are concentrated by your outer ears travel down the ear canal to the eardrum (also called the tympanic membrane).

The tympanic membrane is only about four cell layers thick and less than one quarter inch in diameter. The energy in the sound wave vibrates the tympanic membrane and is mechanically transferred to the inner ear (cochlea) through the three tiny ear bones (also called the ear ossicles). The three tiny ossicles are called the malleus, incus and stapes bones. These bones have descriptive names:

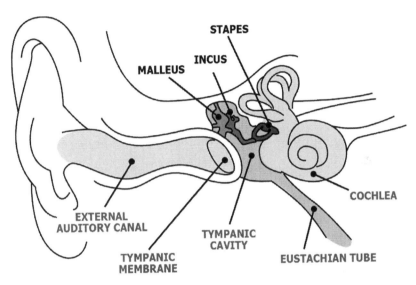

Diagram 1

Malleus "Hammer Bone" – shaped like a tiny farrier's hammer which connects the tympanic membrane to the incus.

Incus "Anvil Bone" – looks like the metal instrument used to shape horseshoes using a farrier's hammer and heat source for the metal. It connects the malleus bone to the stapes bone.

Stapes "Stirrup Bone" – looks like a stirrup on a horse's saddle. It connects the incus to the inner ear through an opening called the oval window. The stapes bone is the smallest bone in the human body!

When sound waves of various frequencies vibrate the tympanic membrane, the sound energy travels from the tympanic membrane through the malleus bone, through the incus bone, through the stapes bone, through the oval window and into the inner ear (also called the cochlea). The inner ear is shaped like a snail shell and has one and three-quarter turns.

 Endolymph [en-d*uh*-limf]
A special fluid contained in the inner ear.

 Cochlea [kok-lee-*uh*, koh-klee-*uh*]
The part of the inner ear that contains a specialized membrane and endolymph fluid.

 Vestibular [ve-stib-y*uh*-ler]
The part of the inner ear that is also called the labrynthine system and regulates balance.

 Tympanic [tim-pan-ik] **membrane**
Commonly known as the ear drum, it conducts sounds from the environment and transfers it to ossicles.

 Ossicles [os-i-k*uh* l]
The three tiny bones in the middle ear that conduct sound energy.

I am going to limit my discussion here to the cochlea. I will discuss more on the vestibular system in a later chapter, as it relates to hearing loss in a condition called "Ménière's syndrome."

In the cochlea, there is a membrane made of specialized cells that travels its entire length. It is here that the mechanical sound vibrations are transformed to electrical impulses. This membrane is arranged tonotopically, meaning that certain areas are dedicated for low frequency sounds (20 – 750Hz), mid-range sounds (800 – 1500Hz) and high-frequency sounds (2000 – 8000 Hz). In the inner ear, the mechanical energy of sound waves is transformed into electrical nerve impulses that then travel through the auditory nerve (also called the acoustic nerve or cranial nerve #8) to the brainstem and subsequently to the temporal lobe area of the brain. Although the tympanic membrane is only 8mm in diameter, its area is about 22 times larger than the stapes bone footplate which connects to the oval window. The difference between the area of the footplate of the stapes and the area of the tympanic membrane results in a huge bio-mechanical advantage and increases sound pressure and energy transfer.

I have always been curious how the cochlea is tonotopically arranged. Looking at Diagram 1, the cochlea has a wide portion at the base and a much narrower portion at the top (apex). Scientists have mapped the cochlea and have found that the wider base area is responsible for high frequency hearing and the narrower apex area is responsible for low frequency hearing. This has never quite made sense to me.

The cochlea's arrangement is actually very important to how we hear. The base of the cochlea is the closest to the outside world and the apex of the cochlea is covered by very dense bone called the petrous (which is Latin for rock) portion of the temporal bone. Since the tympanic membrane is very thin (like tissue paper) it doesn't provide much protection for damage to the inner ear from today's loud sounds in our environment, such as – industrial noise, firearms, rock music, military noise, equipment noise, digital music players with ear buds, etc. This is why loud noise exposure tends to damage high frequencies of hearing easily and the low frequencies of hearing, which are relatively protected by the dense surrounding bone, tend to be preserved well into old age.

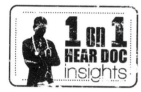 During my junior high school years I played the trumpet in the school marching band. I will never forget marching in the Chicago St. Patrick's Day parade that year, with the Chicago River flowing by (which was dyed green), and seemingly everyone in Chicago waving and cheering as the band played and marched past. In the band, the larger brass instruments like the tubas and baritones produced low sounds and the smaller brass instruments, like my trumpet and the coronets, produced much higher sounds. With this in mind, when I first learned about the anatomy of the cochlea in ENT residency, it was difficult for me to grasp the tonotopical arrangement of the cochlea.

A common hearing problem.

If you have sensorineural hearing loss you may always know when someone is talking to you but you may not always understand what is being said. This is a very common problem. It relates to a pattern of high frequency hearing loss. The low frequencies are usually well preserved throughout life. The sounds of speech which are low frequency are the vowel sounds "a, e, i, o, u." These sounds help you identify speech from other noises. The high-frequency sounds of speech are the constants, especially the fricatives (produced by forcing air through the lips or the teeth). These are sounds such as "sh, th, z, c, s...." They are higher energy and are usually the first areas of the inner ear to be lost in patients with sensorineural hearing loss. These high tones are critical for speech comprehension. Most people with hearing loss can easily identify when someone is speaking (by hearing the low frequencies) but usually cannot understand what is being said (without hearing the high frequencies).

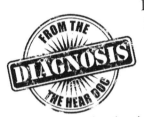

In my practice, I often compare the effects of loud noise to the inner ear to the effects of extremely bright lights, like sunshine, to our vision. Both can be very harmful. Sun exposure can destroy the retinal cells and be quite harmful to vision in the same way that loud noise can harm our hearing. I always encourage patients, regardless of how much hearing loss is present, to wear hearing protection at all times when exposed to loud noise to protect and preserve whatever hearing is left.

There are tens of thousands of veterans with military-service-connected hearing loss, usually due to noise exposure or injuries (such as blasts). For many years, the VA system has supplied hearing aids for these hearing disabled veterans. Until 1994, however, usually only one hearing aid was provided. The researchers devised an ingenious study to see if two hearing aids were required or if just one would suffice. Prior to fitting the standard one hearing aid, they measured both the hearing and the understanding ability (speech discrimination scores) in both ears of each patient. Then they fit one hearing aid (monoaural). The patients were encouraged to wear the hearing aid daily and, after one year, the researchers measured each patient's hearing levels and speech discrimination scores in both ears. What they found was very important. In the aided ear (the ear in which the hearing aid was worn) the speech discrimination scores were *maintained* at the same level from one year prior, but in the unaided ear there was a significant *decrease* in the speech understanding scores.

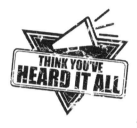

You have heard the phrase "use it or lose it." Well that applies to your hearing as well. You may be wondering if both ears are required for normal hearing or if only one hearing ear can be just as good? That's exactly what a group of researchers working with veterans asked themselves in 1984. Essentially, the researchers found that if you don't stimulate an ear with hearing loss using a hearing aid, you lose hearing ability. As a result of this study and others, in 1994 the VA system began dispensing two hearing aids instead of one to each qualified veteran.

In my ENT office, if a patient insists on only getting one hearing aid, when two would be best, I usually discuss the results of the this study and have the patient sign a waiver that says that although I recommend two hearing aids, the patient only requests one. The loss of understanding ability is avoidable in many patients if hearing aids are obtained soon after the hearing loss is noticed and aids are worn in both ears.

There are several types of hearing loss based on what portion of the ear is not functioning properly.

The first and most common type of hearing loss

 Sensorineural [sen-s*uh*-ree-**n***oo* **r**-*uh* l, -**ny***oo* **r**-]
The most common type of hearing loss associated with the cochlea/nerve (as noted previously).

The second most common type of hearing loss

 Conductive [k*uh* n-**duhk**-tiv]
The type of hearing loss when sounds are not conducted properly from the outer ear to the inner ear (through the ear canal, tympanic membrane and ossicles).

The third most common type of hearing loss

 Mixed [mikst]
This hearing loss is a combination of both conductive and sensorineural hearing losses.

Sudden Sensorineural Hearing Loss (SSHL)

There is another type of hearing loss, which, though not especially common, is very important to recognize and treat. It is called Sudden Sensorineural Hearing Loss (SSHL) and it occurs quite suddenly. I consider sudden sensorineural hearing loss (SSHL) to be a medical emergency. Most cases of SSHL are caused by damage to the inner ear (cochlea) or nerve of hearing. Unfortunately, most commonly the cause is unknown. It can also be associated with vascular disease (a tiny stroke), diabetes, and viral infections.

There are many possible causes of SSHL including:

- head trauma
- skull fracture

- severe loud noise trauma

- ototoxic medications

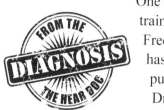

One of my professors during my ENT residency training in Oakland, California, was Dr. Frederick Byl. He is an expert on SSHL, and has studied thousands of cases and has published several studies on the topic. Dr. Byl found that if SSHL occurs with associated dizziness (vertigo), the prognosis (outcome) is poor. However, if no dizziness is associated, there is, generally, a a better chance at regaining some usable hearing, Some patients with SSHL are helped by medical treatment, such as a brief course of high doses of glucocorticoids (steroids). Dr. Byl found that the earlier glucocorticoids are given after the onset of the hearing loss, the better the outcome. He found that in approximately 50% of patients some useful hearing can be regained. I am always concerned when I see patients with SSHL who wait 1-2 months before an ENT evaluation, because the possibility of hearing restoration in these patients requires immediate evaluation and treatment.

I want to briefly mention a rare cause of SSHL. A tumor, called an acoustic neuroma, can grow on the auditory nerve between the cochlea and the brain and result in SSHL, often associated with dizziness and ringing in the ear, but not always. These tumors are almost always benign (not cancerous) and usually grow very slowly, only 1-2 mm per year. A hearing test will often provide clues that this condition is present, like very poor speech discrimination scores in the affected ear, but the best test to diagnose the condition is a magnetic resonance imaging scan (MRI) of the inner ear structures. If an acoustic neuroma is found, treatment has traditionally involved surgical removal (brain surgery), which often results in a total loss of hearing in the affected ear. As with all advances, this procedure has recently become improved. Special radiation treatment, known as "gamma knife," can now focus treatment to these tumors and often stop them from growing, even in some cases shrinking them.

Imagine if you suddenly developed blindness in one eye. Most reasonable people would surely report that same day to their doctor or to an emergency room for urgent evaluation and treatment. How is hearing loss any different?

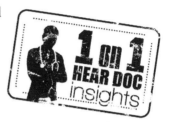

"The louder the better! Loud noise 'toughens up' your hearing and it is not harmful unless it is painful."

FICTION

Noise protection is extremely important to good hearing health. Chronic exposure to loud noise can permanently destroy your hearing and create bothersome tinnitus.

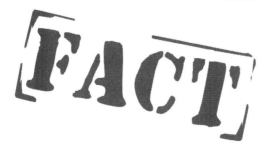

Chapter 4
Hearing Loss Prevention

For tens of thousands of years humans lived on a relatively quiet plant earth, with the exception of loud thunder claps, erupting volcanoes, beating of drums, large waterfalls, the roaring of lions and the sound of other humans yelling.

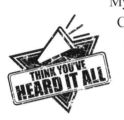

My wife and I used to live in downtown Oakland, California. We loved the weather, the people, the restaurants, the San Francisco Bay, and the diverse variety of weekend activities from which we could choose. At the time, however, we didn't realize how much noise we were constantly exposed to while living there. Our brains had sort of acclimated to a constant barrage of noise and sound pollution. All day long, and usually into the night, we were exposed to noise from auto engines, horns, loud car stereos, diesel city bus engines, construction noise, shopping carts clanging, helicopters, people yelling, delivery vans, etc. About twenty years ago, we were offered a practice opportunity in far northern California and decided to make a change and move to the country. We moved to a home, west of town, in an unincorporated area of grasslands and oak forests on several acres. The difference to our hearing was both immediate and astounding. I will never forget our first night sleeping in our new country home. It was totally quiet; there was no more city noise. Occasionally at night we could hear the train passing through town, but only if the air was humid. The only noise during the day is the blowing of the wind through the window screens, song birds chirping, the occasional cow bellowing and tree leaves rustling. Needless to say, we were pleasantly surprised by the quiet (and I'm sure our hearing has appreciated the change too).

With the industrial revolution and subsequent innovations came the noise that we are exposed to today: engines, machinery, firearms, factories, amplified music, automobiles and thousands of others. Baby Boomers have been exposed to incredibly loud music concerts, personal listening devices, sporting events and other high noise activities. Workplace noise exposure has become more regulated to protect worker hearing and recreational noise exposure is now being recognized in an effort to limit the effect of hearing loss and tinnitus. Did you know that as humans we have built-in noise protection? It is a system of nerves and muscles which attach directly to our eardrums and ear ossicles. Recall, our eardrums are only a few cell layers thick (almost like a piece of paper). The tensor tympani muscle attaches directly to our eardrum and the stapedius muscle attaches to our stapes bone. When a loud noise is present, the muscles contract and stiffen the hearing mechanism to slightly reduce the volume of the sound, this system worked well to protect human hearing prior to industrialization and the noise pollution in today's world.

Stapedial [st*uh*-**pee**-dee-*uh* l] **reflex test**
A test commonly given during a standard audiogram to test the ears natural response to sound protection.

The noises manufactured in our lives today easily overcome your ear's own built in defenses and quickly cause damage. Loud noise does not "toughen up" our hearing, it destroys it. Protecting our ears from those sorts of damaging noises is important.

Noise exposure is generally classified

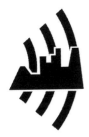

Industrial – examples include:

- Equipment
- Factory Tools
- Machinery noise

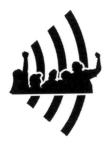

Recreational – examples include:

- Concerts
- Music Players
- Headphones
- Firearm Noise

There are literally thousands of sources of noise in your daily life that can damage your hearing.

In 1971, The United States Occupational Safety and Health Administration (OSHA) formed as an agency of the **United States Department of Labor**. Strict regulations regarding acceptable noise levels were subsequently established to protect workers' hearing. OSHA determined the levels of noise exposure to which you can be safely exposed and prevent permanent hearing damage. The acceptable noise levels are measured in decibels, as well as hours of exposure per day. As you can see from the chart following, if the noise level is less than 85 decibels (dB), there is no limit to the length of exposure without hearing damage, however, noise at any level higher than 90 dB has strict limits to the length of exposure. For example, if the noise level is 100 dB, only 2 hours of noise exposure per day is allowed. At 115 dB, only 15 minutes per day are allowable! If a person is exposed to these levels for longer than the allowed time period per day, hearing protection is needed, usually in the form of ear plugs or ear muffs, or both. In general, ear plugs and ear muffs each reduce the noise exposure by an average of 28 dB. If worn together, there is an additive effect of about 55 dB noise reduction.

PERMISSIBLE NOISE EXPOSURES

HOURS PER DAY	SOUND LEVEL DECIBELS [dB]
8	90
6	92
4	95
3	97
2	100
$1\frac{1}{2}$	102
1	105
$\frac{1}{2}$	110
$\frac{1}{4}$ OR LESS	115

In today's world, as people are exposed to more and more noise on a daily basis, I am seeing permanent hearing loss at younger and younger ages. I recently saw a 13 year old boy who came to the clinic with his mother. 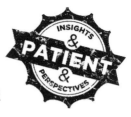 She expressed her concern that the child was not listening to her and felt that he might have hearing loss. There was no family history of deafness and the child had never had ear surgery or frequent ear infections. Her child was however, an avid hunter and target shooter for most of his life. He primarily used shotguns in his right hand and usually without wearing any hearing protection. After a thorough ear exam and audiogram, I found that his recreational activities had resulted in hearing loss in both ears, worse in his left ear (as would be expected with a right handed firearm user), as well as a chronic tinnitus (also worse in the left ear). The test showed bilateral severe sensorineural hearing loss. I discussed my findings with his mother, and told her that his hearing was typical of what we find in an eighty-five year old man's pattern of hearing loss. I then informed her that there was nothing I could do surgically. The mother started crying and sobbing when she heard the news. I explained that the hearing loss could have been prevented completely by the use of hearing protection. I asked the child to always wear hearing protection when using firearms and when exposed to other loud noises to preserve his remaining hearing. I fitted him with two hearing aids, which he subsequently wore. Years later, he is still wearing hearing aids and is still passionate about hunting as he runs his own hunting guide business.

Protect your ears from exposure to these noises

Sound becomes painful to our ears at **about 125-130 dB.**

 rock concert can be as high as 100-130 dB depending on venue size and how close to the speakers you sit.

 gun blast is approximately 160 dB at the muzzle.

 iPods or iPhones with ear buds deliver high sound pressures up to 120 dB. In the European Union, these audio devices come with a built in volume limiter for maximum output of 85-89 dB. (but not in the U.S.)

 an airplane taking off 180 dB

lawnmower 100 dB

 motorcycle 100 dB

firecracker 150 dB

 rocket launch 180 dB

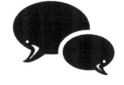

normal conversation

Speaking is about 60 dB.

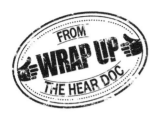

I like to compare the wearing of hearing protection to wearing sunglasses. Just as staring at the sun can damage your vision, exposure to loud noises can damage your hearing. I also firmly believe that it is very important to eat a well-balanced diet, and if necessary, to take supplemental vitamins to ensure that your body has all the nutrients it needs to function properly.

There are several companies that market vitamins to purportedly help your hearing, reduce tinnitus, and prevent hearing loss. I believe that there is some benefit to supplemental vitamins/minerals, particularly if you have a specific condition called "otosclerosis" (addressed in a later chapter). In this condition, it has been shown in several large trials that sodium fluoride supplementation can stabilize formation of the otosclerotic process and slow down the subsequent development of hearing loss, tinnitus and dizziness symptoms in some patients.

"Earwax is dirt and should be removed
from your ears each day or you will
not be able to hear well."

FICTION

Although it is unsightly, earwax
has several protective functions and
should not be routinely cleaned out of the ear,
unless it creates problems.

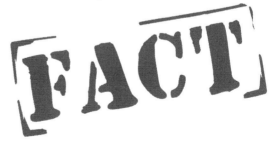

Chapter 5
Earwax: It's Not Dirt!

Earwax (and other things found in the ears)

I could not write a book about hearing and hearing loss without at least a brief chapter on earwax. If you take nothing else away from this chapter, know this: "Earwax is not dirt!" Earwax is essential for a normal functioning ear.

 Cerumen _[si-**roo**-m*uh* n]
The earwax produced by glands in the outer portion of the ear canal skin.

Although it is not very appealing, earwax has many beneficial and valuable properties which protect our ears. Earwax has been found to contain ear infection fighting properties. It is slightly acidic and contains antibodies, both of which have protective functions. It also lubricates and soothes our ear canals, insulates against temperature extremes, repels insects, keeps water and soap out of the ear, and prevents irritation and itching problems. Normally, the earwax migrates naturally to the outside of the ear canal and is eliminated invisibly (similar to the dead skin on the rest of our bodies). Earwax production is influenced by hormones including estrogen. As most people (men and women) age, less estrogen is produced and therefore also less earwax.

Chronic ear canal itching is easily treated by simply leaving a small film of earwax in the canal and by instilling a few drops of white distilled vinegar to re-acidify the ear canal. Of course, there may be a bigger problem causing the itching, such as an infection, so seeing an ENT doctor for evaluation, if it persists, is important.

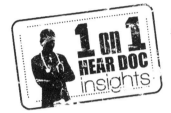

A problem I commonly treat in older (post-menopausal) women is chronic itching of the ear canals. This is usually caused by three factors:

- Decreased earwax production
- Excessive cleaning of the ear canals
- The use of chemical drying agents in the ear canal such as rubbing alcohol or hydrogen peroxide.

Cerumen comes in two types: wet and dry. It is actually a genetically inherited trait. Most people with dry cerumen are of Asian descent and most people with wet cerumen are of African descent. In Europe and the Americas there is a mix of cerumen types. The glands in the ear which produce cerumen are very similar to the glands in women which produce breast milk. Some research has even shown a higher breast cancer risk in women with wet cerumen versus dry cerumen.

Many of my patients apologize to me prior to their ear examination for having "dirty ears" when actually the opposite is true. Earwax is not dirt and when present usually indicates a healthy ear canal. Sometimes it is necessary for me to remove earwax to examine the deeper ear structures. Earwax production shuts down during ear infections as the earwax glands go into shock from the infections. Of course, too much earwax can cause problems including hearing loss.

Impacted Cerumen [si-**roo**-m*uh* n]
The buildup of excessive earwax in the ear.

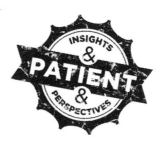

I am constantly amazed with the ingenuity I see in my office from patients attempting to remove earwax from their ear canals. They tend to use almost any small object which may be handy, such as:

- Bobby Pins
- Fingers & Fingernails
- Nails
- Screws
- Toothpicks
- Matches
- Blunt end of utensils
- Various other small, sharp objects

Needless to say, the use of these objects is dangerous and often produces infection. Moreover, these approaches usually don't get the job done anyway.

Others resort to the use of "ear candling." This is a trend in which a special "earwax removing" candle or cone is lit on fire and inserted into the ear canal. As a physician, I do not recommend this practice. Not only is there a risk of fire or burns to the hair and face, but there are reports of house fires and even one death associated with this kind of candle use. Scientific studies have shown that this process does not result in significant removal of earwax.

Of course "Q-tips" are most often used, however Q-tips are about the same width as the average ear canal and when they are inserted into the ear, can frequently push the earwax from the outer canal (where it is formed) into the deeper portion of the ear canal next to the tympanic membrane. This can result in worsened hearing loss and impacted cerumen which usually requires removal by a medical professional. The old saying "Don't put anything in your ear smaller than your elbow" is actually good advice if you want to avoid outer ear problems. In general, your ears do not need routine cleaning in any area not accessible by a wash cloth and attempts to "clean" the ears by other means often produce problems.

Ear irrigation

Many physicians have their nurse irrigate a patient's ears with a large metal syringe filled with warm water. This is a messy process, so usually a basin is placed under the ear to collect the water and cerumen. Although this process is usually safe, unfortunately I have seen many problems including laceration and bruising of the ear canal, infections and even rupture and perforation of the tympanic membrane with hearing loss. I have had to surgically repair tympanic membranes, in the past, due to complications from ear irrigation.

I usually use a high-powered surgical microscope to easily access and remove earwax with a small wire loop or tiny forceps. I generally do not use water irrigation to remove earwax. I am thrilled when I am able to quickly and painlessly remove impacted cerumen resulting in happy patients with immediately improved hearing and relief of symptoms.

In 1994, I spent a one month ENT externship in a large metropolitan hospital in the Los Angeles area. During that month, I saw several patients in the emergency room with foreign bodies in their ears. The patients were usually adults and the foreign objects were usually live cockroaches! The typical patient came into the ER Screaming "Get it out !!" When the ER attending physician called me down to help, the first thing I would do is flood the ear with liquid lidocaine anesthetic. This immediately paralyzed the insect and provided instant relief to the patient. I usually used the surgical microscope and micro forceps to remove the insect and solve the problem. Those patients were the most grateful patients I have ever seen. I'm sure I got a few appreciative hugs afterwards. I don't think that the insect problem could have been prevented with a little earwax, but maybe it would have protected the ear enough for the bugs to go elsewhere!

There is an over-the-counter earwax removal kit that I like which includes some earwax softening drops and a small irrigation bulb, which is used to gently irrigate the ear canal with warm water. It works fairly well and I sometimes recommend it if there is no history of previous ear surgery or infection. It is marketed under the name "Murine Ear Cleaning Kit" and costs about $20.

The skin of the ear canal has almost no fat tissue to pad the nerves on the underlying bone. Because of this, earwax removal can be quite uncomfortable. With the microscope and my tiny surgical instruments like curettes and "alligator" forceps, I can usually very comfortably remove the earwax from my patient's ears and barely touch the sensitive ear canal skin. There are 4 different nerves which supply sensation to the ear canal. One of these is called the Vagus nerve, which is also called cranial nerve #10. The nerve is called the Vagus from the Latin "vagrant" because it literally wanders throughout the body. It has branches to the ears, nose, throat, heart, lungs and intestines. The branch to the ear is sometimes called "Arnold's nerve." Stimulation of this nerve during ear cleaning can sometimes elicit a brief coughing reflex in certain patients.

When I remove patient's earwax in my office, I tend to use my Zeiss German surgical microscope *(pictured to right)*. Using the microscope, the ear canal structures are clearly magnified and any earwax problems are easy to see.

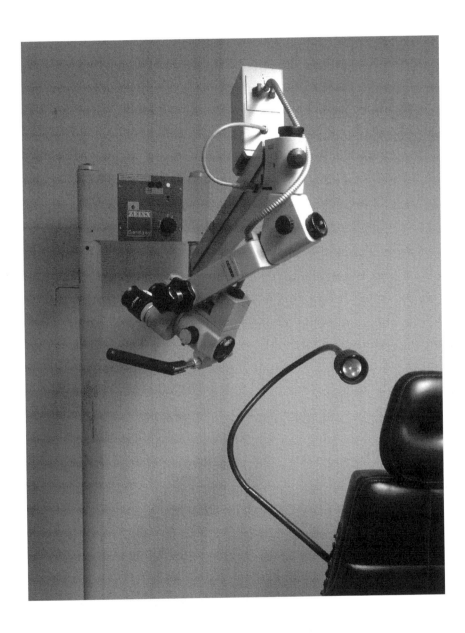

"If I had a hearing loss, my family doctor would have told me."

FICTION

Very few primary care givers routinely measure your hearing; therefore, it is virtually impossible for most doctors to recognize your hearing loss, unless it is advanced.

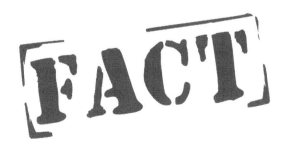

SECTION 2
Tests - Audiogram and Ear Exam

This section covers everything you need to know about hearing testing and alternatives to hearing aids that are sometimes worth considering. It is important that the first thing you do is to have a microscopic ear exam and a complete diagnostic audiogram. Both of these procedures are brief and painless and typically take 25-30 minutes each. These procedures should be completed by your local board-certified ENT physician. Why is that so important? Because the testing will yield a wealth of information that will ensure the right treatment decisions are made. If you think that you may have a hearing loss, schedule these simple tests. The results may be eye-opening.

The following topics will be covered in this section:
- When is it important to see an ear physician?
- The steps and procedures of a hearing test/exam
- What is that ringing sound in your ears?
- Alternatives to restoring hearing without using aids.

"There is nothing that can be done about the ringing in your ears, so you must learn to live with it."

FICTION

Ringing in the ears is successfully treated in over 90% of patients using a combination of methods including avoidance of certain medications, surgical procedures, biofeedback, specially designed hearing aids, and herbal remedies.

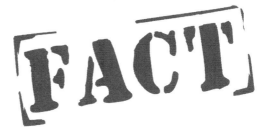

Chapter 6
Ringing in the Ears (Tinnitus)

Almost all of us have experienced at some time in our lives a ringing sound in our ears. You may have experienced it after exposure to loud noise in the environment around you, such as loud concerts, engine noise, or firearms. This ringing sound can also occur for other reasons, like taking certain medications (even aspirin) or perhaps during a very stressful time in your life. The sound in your head is called tinnitus. The word is derived from the Latin word for ringing. Tinnitus has two possible pronunciations as either ti-NIGHT-us or TIN-it-us depending on which dictionary you read. Most ENT physicians I know including myself, prefer the latter.

 Tinnitus (ti-NIGHT-us or TIN-i-tus)

The perception of sound when no sound is present.

Tinnitus can be medically characterized in two manners:

- **Subjective tinnitus** is only heard by the patient
- **Objective tinnitus** can be heard by others (rare)

Tinnitus is further characterized in the following types:

- **Continuous tinnitus** - the most common form
- **Pulsatile tinnitus** - may indicate a bigger problem

Tinnitus can be very distressing. It is often a constant sound and can be particularly bothersome at night. It is usually present in both ears but can also occur in only one ear. It is estimated that over 30 million people in the U.S. suffer from this condition. When it is uncomfortable to patients, they will sometimes mention the problem to their primary care physician who will usually respond in the following manner, "There is nothing you can do about it, so you'll have to just live with it."

In my years of practice, I have heard patients use many different comparisons to describe the tinnitus sound that they hear in their head. If I describe your experience, I'm here to tell you there is almost always something that can be done about tinnitus.

Tinnitus can sound like:

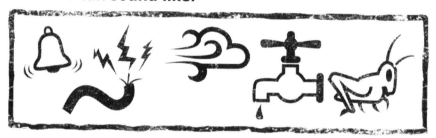

- Crickets
- Roaring
- Blowing
- Ocean type noises
- High tension electric wire noise

- Clicking
- Ringing
- Musical sounds
- Bells
- Leaky faucet

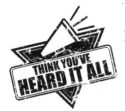

I have only heard objective tinnitus in two patients in my entire career thus far. I have a special instrument called a Toynbee tube which is essentially a stethoscope with an earpiece on the other end. In both of the patients, they described a bothersome clicking sound in only one ear. I told them that I may be able to hear the sounds in their heads as well and they laughed in disbelief. I asked them to hold their breath to eliminate the breathing sounds and inserted the listening end of my Toynbee tube into the affected ear. I was not sure if I would actually hear anything, but to my surprise I could hear the sounds that the patients had been concerned about.

In pulsatile tinnitus, a patient is usually hearing his/her own blood flow. It may be the flow from the heart (arterial) or back to the heart (venous). Pulsatile tinnitus can be caused by a tumor (which can occasionally be cancerous) in the middle ear or by an abnormally large blood vessel. There are some high-tech imaging tests which can be performed such as an MRI or MRA (magnetic resonance arteriography) or angiography to identify these rare tumors. I most commonly see pulsatile tinnitus in women who have had multiple pregnancies (multiparous). During pregnancy, the blood volume in a woman's body increases significantly and can stretch out the veins, including the veins in the middle ear and occasionally, as a result of this, the increased blood flow can be heard.

If the patient has allergies, this can also cause tinnitus, so I also perform allergy skin testing and start them on an allergy treatment protocol.

Another interesting cause of tinnitus is Ménière's syndrome. It is a clinical syndrome which affects only one ear about 85% of the time and both ears about 15% of the time. The tinnitus in Ménière's syndrome is usually described as a "rushing" or "roaring" sound, and it is usually associated with a low-frequency sensorineural hearing loss, a sensation of "fullness" in the affected ear, and can cause episodes of severe vertigo and dizziness. Ménière's syndrome's cause is unknown, but it results in too much inner ear fluid. It is made much worse by high-salt (sodium) diets, alcohol, allergies, caffeine, large meals and certain medications. When I see a patient with Ménière's syndrome, the first thing I ask them is whether they have had any recent dietary changes which may include higher sodium intake.

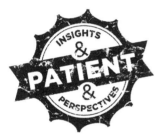

During my residency, I remember treating a 32 year-old patient who had multiple pregnancies and subsequently developed a very bothersome venous pulsatile tinnitus in one ear. When I examined her ears, she had completely normal results and her hearing tests revealed no problems. However, when I gently compressed her jugular vein on the side of the tinnitus, the sound completely disappeared until I released the compression. Her imaging study was negative for a tumor. I discussed the findings with the Chief ENT doctor and because the problem caused this patient much discomfort, and as an experiment with her consent, we decided to tie off the jugular vein on that side. When this is done, the other jugular vein takes care of the blood flow from both sides. Immediately after surgery her tinnitus was cured and she no longer heard the pulsation. The patient was elated with the results! She continued to have excellent results for about one week, however unfortunately the tinnitus returned roughly 7 days after the procedure. The patient's body had quickly re-established the blood flow. Because of this, I haven't performed this procedure since.

I usually tell patients to avoid prepared foods such as canned goods, cheese, processed meats, and especially fast foods, which can be extremely high in sodium. I also encourage patients to avoid alcoholic beverages, caffeine, and to eat smaller portions of food more frequently, to avoid a high sodium load all at once. If none of these measures are working to control the tinnitus or other symptoms of Ménière's, I will sometimes start the patient on a diuretic (water pill) to try and flush the extra sodium through the kidneys. If diuretics fail to control the symptoms of Ménière's, there are several other, much more invasive treatments, including surgical procedures, which can be performed.

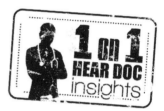

One of the biggest culprits related to Ménière's syndrome that I have seen is dietary weight loss plans that include prepared meals, as they tend to come loaded with high sodium content. The first step in the treatment of Ménière's is to stress safety precautions to prevent accidents and injury from the vertigo episodes (if present). The second step in treatment is a low sodium diet. There are some great low sodium dietary tips available online at various websites.

The most common type of tinnitus is a continuous sound which is heard in both ears. It is usually described as a high pitched ringing sound and is almost always subjective rather than objective. The patient usually says it is worse at night or when they are in a very quiet room. Occasionally it has been known to be louder than the patient's own voice. In these cases, the patient is usually quite distressed or even depressed because of it. I have found that when high-pitched tinnitus is present there is often an associated high-frequency sensorineural hearing loss. There is a great test in addition to the standard audiogram for these patients. It is called the "tinnitus matching test." This test provides a good idea of how the patient hears the tinnitus, including the frequency and perceived loudness. It is usually between 4000 Hz and 8000Hz and 5 or 10 dB louder than their hearing thresholds and tends to align the high frequency sensorineural hearing loss at the same frequency as the tinnitus matching. This matching test gives ENT physicians helpful information to determine the best treatment.

There are several things that can cause or worsen tinnitus. As I just mentioned, it is commonly an associated high frequency hearing loss. Many over-the-counter medications can cause or worsen existing tinnitus, products like aspirin, Pepto Bismol, and Alka Seltzer, which may contain salicylates, the group name drugs of this type. Of course, aspirin is also a powerful medication to help prevent heart attacks, so I usually do not recommend that patients discontinue aspirin products without first speaking to their primary care physician about the risks and benefits of aspirin therapy.

Other common factors that contribute to making tinnitus worse are nicotine, caffeine, increased stress, depression, and TMJ (jaw joint arthritis). Nicotine and caffeine are stimulants and I always advise patients to quit smoking or chewing tobacco, whether or not they have tinnitus. Doing so can also help to reduce symptoms of tinnitus. I also advise patients to discontinue caffeine containing products or at least switch to half-caffeinated beverages to decrease their caffeine consumption. I have found that patients who feel they have lots of life stress more commonly suffer the worst tinnitus symptoms. Usually when they go away on a stress-free vacation, the tinnitus is less noticeable or absent. In this case, I often counsel patients to reduce their current stress level as much as possible. This can be achieved in a variety of ways:

- Picking up a relaxing hobby

- Meditating

- Exercise

- Biofeedback methods

- Stress-relieving medications

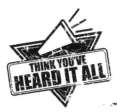

When severe, tinnitus can cause depression and in some patients, depression can cause tinnitus (thus it becomes a vicious cycle). Interestingly enough, one long accepted treatment for tinnitus is anti-depressant medications, which has had some success in the treatment of my patients. I saw one patient with tinnitus that was so severe that it had resulted in major depression to the point where the patient was actually considering suicide. I immediately referred him for professional psychiatric care. Fortunately, tinnitus is rarely this severe – but it is important to mention if you feel that way. You are not alone – and there are doctors and other professionals to help.

There is another option to treat tinnitus called tinnitus retraining therapy (TRT). This treatment can take many months and is usually done on a one-to-one basis. Its purpose is not necessarily to reduce or eliminate the tinnitus, but to train the brain to ignore the sound and push it to the background. It can be very successful in a highly motivated patient.

If you are looking for other relief remedies there are several over-the-counter options to curb the irritation of tinnitus. Most are herbal remedies which are sprayed into the nose, taken orally or placed as drops into the ear canal. These products may contain several different herbal substances, vitamins or minerals and can be effective in some patients to reduce tinnitus. These products are not regulated by the FDA.

Finally, there is a wonderful organization that has helped thousands of patients with tinnitus. It is called the American Tinnitus Association *(ATA)* – **www.ata.org**

Tinnitus is not something you must live with. It can be successfully treated in most patients. Tinnitus is a very common disorder which is usually mild, but can occasionally be severe and produce significant discomfort. It can be measured by a simple audiology test called

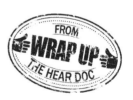

tinnitus matching. Tinnitus usually has associated hearing loss, but not always. It is worsened by aspirin products, nicotine, caffeine, stress, TMJ problems and depression. There is almost always something that can be done to help tinnitus, including discontinuation of certain medications, discontinuation of nicotine and caffeine, use of special hearing aids, biofeedback, life stress reduction, treatment of depression, tinnitus retraining therapy and herbal remedies.

....

"I can't bear the silent ringing in my skull."

-Jonathan Lethem

....

ENT physicians are expensive and they will just push their own hearing aid products, so I might as well go to a hearing aid shop.

FICTION

A well-staffed ENT physician's office is your one-stop-shop for everything to do with your ears; from ear cleaning, ear surgery, medical treatment, testing of your hearing, to hearing aid dispensing.

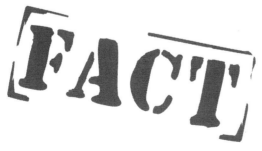

Chapter 7

The Importance of Seeing an ENT Physician

Why is it important to see an ENT Physician? There are only about 225 new board-certified ENT physicians trained each year for the entire population of the United States, which at the time of this writing is approximately 350 million people. That's about one new ENT physician for every 1.5 million people per year. There are currently about 10,500 ENT doctors practicing in the U.S. I am one of those board-certified ENT physicians (a.k.a. otolaryngologist) with many years of college, medical school and postgraduate education. In case you didn't know, this medical specialty is the oldest in the U.S.

There is a developing trend in the U.S. where each year, more ENT physicians are dispensing hearing aids. This is a fortunate development for people who suffer from hearing loss. The reason for this is simple; an ENT physician knows a lot about the ear and hearing loss and is an excellent choice for treatment of hearing loss and ear conditions.

In the U.S., audiologists can also be licensed to sell hearing aids. They typically have 6-8 years of college and usually have a Master's degree or a Doctor of Audiology degree. There are currently about 12,800 audiologists practicing in the U.S. as of 2009.

A hearing aid dispenser who is not an audiologist or physician or even medically trained, can also become licensed to sell hearing aids with only a high school diploma. Each state has different hearing aid dispenser licensing requirements, but usually it consists of a 1-2 hour written exam and a half-day practical exam. In some states it is required to spend several weeks training with an audiologist or an ENT physician, before being able to dispense on their own. Most hearing aid dispensers learn "on-the-job" or are supervised by another hearing aid dispenser, thus, a formal educational requirement is not typically expected.

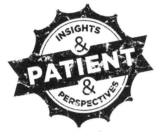

In 1995, I was a young ENT physician, having recently completed my five year ENT physician residency training program, and had been practicing in Northern California for only about a year. At that time, I had been referring all my patients with hearing loss, who I could not help with surgery or medical treatment, for hearing aids to an audiologist in a nearby town about 30 miles away. One day a patient asked me why she had to travel out of the area to obtain quality hearing aids. She then asked, "Dr. Frantz, why can't you sell hearing aids?" Her question made me start thinking that maybe I should incorporate hearing aid dispensing into my practice. About a month later, I received a telephone call from an ENT physician colleague in Sacramento, California. He said, "Frantz, this is your lucky day!" When I asked, "Why?" he replied, "My hearing aid dispenser's husband is moving to your area to work at the bottling plant and she is moving up with him and is looking for an ENT physician to work with and dispense hearing aids." Shortly after our conversation, I had a new audiologist working with me! To legally dispense hearing aids in my practice, I also had to study and obtain a hearing aid dispensing license, and that is how I started helping many more people hear better with hearing aids than I could ever help with surgery.

Now that you have the knowledge, ask yourself who you think is best qualified to diagnose and treat your hearing loss? Of course I am biased, but I believe ENT physicians are uniquely qualified. Not only can an ENT physician perform a complete

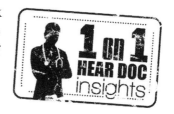

physical exam (usually with a surgical microscope) to provide a diagnosis of the cause for your hearing loss (which may not just be your ears), but an ENT physician can also:

- Remove earwax
- Perform hearing restoration surgery
- Prescribe medications
- Dispense hearing aids if needed

Hopefully, by now you have a better understanding about how important hearing is, how we hear, and what can go wrong with our hearing. You have also had a glimpse into my ENT physician experience, and you know about some of the most common ear conditions that an ENT treats. The next crucial step for you to take is to schedule an evaluation with a hearing professional. As I have mentioned previously, I strongly believe that the most important step in evaluation of your ears and hearing is to see an ENT first. Regardless of whether or not you have insurance coverage to have specialty ENT physician care, look at it as an investment in your hearing (costs for the complete evaluation are typically between $175 - $350). Some private health insurance carriers require a referral from your primary care provider prior to seeing an ENT specialist; however in most cases

Medicare insurance covers ENT physician specialty care without a referral from your primary care physician. If the ENT orders a diagnostic audiogram to further evaluate your hearing or to evaluate further conditions such as tinnitus, vertigo or chronic ear infections, the audiogram charges are also usually covered by Medicare and most private insurances. However, if the audiogram is performed solely for the purpose of obtaining hearing aids, the costs may not be covered by Medicare.

If you have any of the following conditions, in many cases, hearing can be restored by an ENT physician using medication or simple in-office procedures – thus an ENT evaluation is extremely important. These include a history of ear infections, previous ear surgery, ear "tube" insertions, sudden deafness, ear pain, vertigo, ringing in your ears, ear drainage, impacted ear wax, deformity of the ear, Ménière's Syndrome, a family history of hearing loss, ototoxic medications (i.e. some types of chemotherapy for cancer), neurosurgery, head trauma, perforated eardrum, bleeding from the ear, growths in the ear canal, ear itching, or sensitive hearing.

Due to increasing demands on physicians with government regulations (Affordable Care Act or "Obamacare"), computerized medical records and declining insurance reimbursements, many older ENT physicians are retiring prematurely from practice. This has led to a relative shortage of ENT physicians nationwide. According to the American Academy of Otolaryngology (ENT) approximately 59% of counties in the United States do NOT have a practicing, board-certified ENT physician. If you are fortunate enough to have an ENT in your town, schedule an appointment for a complete history and examination of your ears and hearing. An ENT physician will not only perform a complete ear examination, perform surgical procedures, treat medical ear conditions and evaluate you for industrial noise induced hearing loss, but they will also give you the most experienced and expert advice on how to best help you hear better.

According to a 2009 Consumer Reports study, the best place to purchase hearing aids is from an ENT physician who employs an audiologist that fits and dispenses hearing aids. Medicare usually covering the cost of the ENT physician's examination and the audiologist's hearing testing, especially if the visit is not exclusively to get hearing aids.

An ENT physician is best qualified to treat hearing loss. As previously mentioned, audiologists and hearing aid dispensers can also treat hearing loss, but can only help your hearing by providing hearing aids.

I will also caution you that there is a huge retail markup in price for hearing aids. Don't be fooled by full-page newspaper advertisements or fancy color direct mailers advertising for:

- Hearing Aid Discounts
- Buy One Get One Free
- 50% off MSRP (Manufacturer's Suggested Retail Price)
- FREE Video Ear Evaluation
- 3 Days Only Open House

Although these advertisements may be perfectly legal in your state, the only purpose of the ads is to get you to go into a dispenser's hearing aid sales office so they can sell you some hearing aids (think of it like going to car lot). The price markup and hidden costs are there to recoup the huge marketing budget spent and is not a reflection of the sophisticated or un-sophisticated make up of your hearing aid. Trust your hearing to a physician. In most ENT offices, hearing aid sales are provided as an ancillary service for their patients and ENT physicians are not dependent on hearing aid sales to pay the bills. Let me repeat that: ENT physicians' businesses are not dependent on selling hearing aids! It is an ancillary service to help make it easier for you. There is usually much less pressure to purchase hearing aids. ENT physicians simply want to help their patients improve their hearing, whether it's with surgery, medications or with the use of hearing aids.

In the U.S., the hearing aid sales law states that any patient under the age of 18 years of age MUST first be evaluated by a physician prior to purchasing hearing aids. Anyone over the age of 18 years must sign a waiver to a physician's examination prior to purchasing hearing aids. The other option is to be examined and cleared for hearing aid use by a physician prior to purchasing hearing aids from a non-physician (audiologist or hearing aid dispenser). The law requires that patients intending to buy hearing aids must either have a medical exam or sign a waiver saying they do not want a medical exam to rule out a medical reason for their hearing loss before buying hearing aids. The U.S. FDA (Food and Drug Administration) believes that it is in your best health interest to have a medical examination by a licensed physician, preferably one that specializes in ear diseases, before buying hearing aids. I don't know the specific reason(s) why the FDA passed this law, but I assume that it was to protect you, the consumer, from harm and to help ensure that patients with hearing loss have the best care possible, and truly need hearing aids. In 5-10 % of patients with hearing loss, medical and/or surgical treatment by a physician (preferably an ENT) can restore hearing without the use of hearing aids.

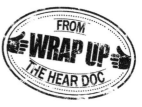

My recommendation is: don't sign any sort of waiver or medical agreement without visiting an ENT physician and get the best possible care for your ears and hearing. If there is no ENT available or for some reason you decide not to see an ENT for your hearing loss, be extremely wary if earwax removal is recommended to be performed by the hearing aid dispenser or audiologist. If earwax removal is suggested, make sure the individual is qualified and licensed to do so. Ask to see his/her training credentials in your state.

Unfortunately, I frequently see injuries from earwax removal by well-meaning hearing aid providers and nurses, who are just not as experienced or professionally trained to do this procedure. I have seen many serious conditions that have resulted from various providers trying to remove earwax. These distressful conditions include bleeding from the ear canal, extreme pain, ruptured ear drums, worsened hearing loss and serious infections. Many of these patients have needed me to perform corrective surgery to restore their hearing and repair the damage. As I stated earlier, earwax is not dirt -- earwax present in your ear canal actually creates a healthier ear canal. However, earwax removal is often a necessary procedure in order for an ENT physician to perform a complete examination of the ear drum or to perform an ear impression, necessary for a custom hearing aid. Laws vary from state to state covering who can legally and safely remove earwax from your ear. In California, for example, physicians, physician assistants, family nurse practitioners, nurses (under a doctor's supervision), and audiologists can remove earwax. Hearing aid dispensers cannot.

Not all ENT physicians care for ears and hearing. An increasing number of my colleagues practice in ENT subspecialties such as Head and Neck Cancer, Pediatric, Rhinology (nasal expert), and Facial Plastic Surgery. Before you schedule an appointment with an ENT make sure that he/she performs ear and hearing evaluations. You may also want to ask if the ENT has any audiologists or hearing aid dispensers who work with him/her in the office for complete continuity of your hearing care. If you don't know which ENT physician is in your insurance network, simply go to the company's website and search by specialty, doctor's name or zip code to find a participating ENT or call the telephone number on the back of your insurance card.

....

"The most basic of all human needs is the need to understand and to be understood. The best way to understand people is to listen to them."

-Ralph G. Nichols

....

Hearing tests are lengthy, uncomfortable procedures done in smelly sound chambers, and take hours to complete.

FICTION

The audiogram is a simple, painless test of your hearing done by an ENT, audiologist or hearing aid dispenser in a special quiet room and usually takes only 15-20 minutes to complete.

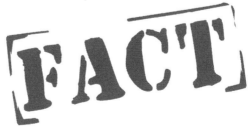

Chapter 8
The Hearing Test (Audiogram)

So now you have found a qualified ENT physician and are ready to get a hearing test. Unlike other medical tests, a hearing test is simple and painless. There are no needles, no fasting is required, and there is no need to "prep" your body in any way; you just need to show up (although you should avoid loud noise for at least 8 hours prior).

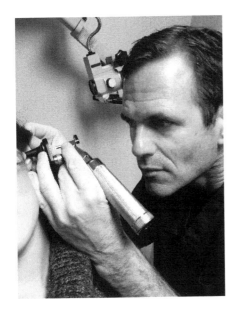

Patient having ear examination by Dr. Frantz.

When they arrive in my clinic, my patients complete a simple questionnaire which is called the **"Hearing Health Assessment"** *(presented in Section 1: Chapter 2).* If a patient responds "Yes" to any of the 10 questions, I perform a complete ENT evaluation prior to any hearing testing. It helps to focus the hearing test components for a more accurate diagnosis. However, even if a patient responds "No" to all 10 hearing health questions, prior to anyone having a hearing test, the ears must be examined. I look for any obstructions of the ear canals or other medical conditions, such as ear infection, which may need treatment prior to the hearing testing.

There are many different ways to test hearing. The simplest hearing test is a forced whisper from across the examination room. It is not very accurate, but can give a gauge on the severity of the potential hearing loss. Another test is the "finger rub" where I simply rub my thumb and index fingers together fairly close to the patient's ear as I ask if they hear it. This is slightly more accurate.

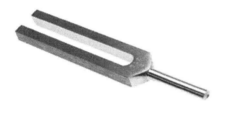

For decades physicians have tested hearing with tuning forks. These are metal objects with two tines (like a fork) that vibrate at various frequencies. These are the same instruments used to tune pianos, hence the name. The most common tuning fork frequency used to test hearing is 512 Hz, which is middle "C" on a piano. I also use 1024 Hz and 2048 Hz tuning forks. I feel that the tuning fork provides much more accurate hearing testing than the whispered voice or the finger rub.

The most accurate hearing test is called a diagnostic audiogram. An audiogram is a comprehensive test of your hearing ability and is composed of a battery of simple tests. I will describe the process, in detail, shortly.

Audiogram [aw-dee-*uh*-gram]
A visually graphic representation of the hearing findings, presented in a chart or graph format.

The graph usually has loudness spanning vertically (on the Y-axis) and various frequency tones horizontally displayed (on the X-axis). Speech testing is generally also performed using either the tester's voice or recorded speech.

I also commonly test the health of the tympanic membrane and middle ears using gentle pressure through a computer probe in each ear. This is called a tympanogram. My office has a computerized hearing testing device that does not require any response on the part of the patient. It is especially great for testing children's hearing and is called "otoacoustic emissions" (OAE) testing. I can test 12 different frequencies with our current equipment. The basis of OAEs requires a much more lengthy discussion and explanation and is beyond the scope of this book.

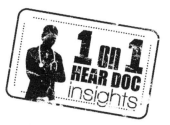

To ensure an accurate hearing test, a quiet test environment is required. Although some hearing professionals simply use a quiet room, I prefer to test in a sound booth. The sound booth is acoustically manufactured to reduce external noise and provide the most accurate audiogram. It is generally not a soundproof room, but a sound shielded room. They are well ventilated. The booths are usually constructed of insulated, perforated steel, usually with a window or two so the examiner can see the patient's responses during the test and so the patient feels comfortable and not claustrophobic.

If you have had a hearing test already, you know what I'm talking about. Our booths are quite large and occupy an entire examination room. The examiner site is outside the booth where most of the test equipment is located. Many ENT offices have a sound booth and audiology testing equipment. My ENT office has a sound booth, and I try to make it a pleasant experience with new carpeting, comfortable seating, air fresheners and good ventilation.

Once you are seated in the sound booth to perform the audiogram, either a headset or ear canal insert speakers are used. A series of pure tones (beeping sounds) are triggered at several different frequencies and are presented to each of your ears. In order to get an accurate test, it is very important that no matter how soft the tone may sound to you, you should respond. If you even think you heard it you should indicate a response to the examiner. We are professionals, and as experts, you will not confuse the hearing examiners if you respond too much. A score for each frequency is actually marked at the sound level at which you respond 50% of the time.

A special test of your bone conduction hearing is then performed. A bone vibration instrument is placed somewhere on your head and the sounds then travel directly through your skull to the inner ears, bypassing the ear canals and tympanic membranes. If there is a difference between pure tone testing using the headset and the bone conduction, it often means that the patient has either conductive or mixed hearing loss (as discussed in more detail later in this chapter).

When the pure tone testing is completed, speech testing is usually performed. The hearing examiner will instruct you through the headset. During speech testing either a live or recorded voice will be used. Usually several things are tested including:

- **Speech Reception Threshold** (SRT): the loudness level at which you can clearly hear speech.

- **Speech Discrimination** (or understanding ability with amplification)

- **Most Comfortable Level of speech** (MCL)

- **Uncomfortable Level of speech** (UCL)

The last two levels are very important. The difference between MCL and UCL is called the "dynamic range." This range becomes extremely important if you decide to get hearing aids, as this range is the amplification (gain) of the hearing aids which are best for you. If you have a large dynamic range you will be easier to fit with hearing aids and if it is small, the hearing aid fitting may be more difficult because sounds can become uncomfortably loud with very little amplification.

Finally, the tympanogram and occasionally otoacoustic emissions testing is performed. The whole process of the testing may sound complicated, but with an experienced hearing examiner it usually only takes 15-20 minutes. When your hearing test is complete, the audiogram is provided in a hard copy. The graph obtained can be quite complex so make sure your ENT physician or audiologist/dispenser explains it to you.

I take special care with my patients to make sure I answer all their questions before they leave the office (and remember there are no "stupid questions").

Typical Adult Hearing Loss Audiogram Chart View

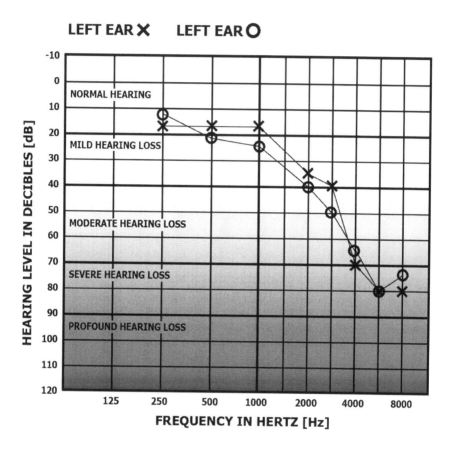

The right and left ears are usually shown separately with one graph for the left ear and one for the right, although sometimes both ears are together on the same graph (as above). The right ear is always represented by a red color or an "O" and the left ear is always represented by a blue color or an "X". Usually the sound levels at which you heard the different tones are located on the vertical axis (y-axis). The different frequencies tested are usually located on the horizontal axis (x-axis).

The sound loudness levels are measured in decibels (dB). The decibel scale of sound measurement is a logarithmic scale, not a linear scale. For example a sound at 20 dB is not twice as loud as a sound at 10 dB; it is 100 times louder.

- **Normal** hearing is generally considered to be at 25 dB or less for each frequency tested.
- **Mild** hearing loss is between 25 dB – 45 dB.
- **Moderately severe** hearing loss is 45 dB – 70 dB.
- **Severe** hearing loss is 70 dB – 90 dB.
- **Profound** hearing loss is over 90 dB, which can often be beyond the limit of the testing equipment.

Normal Hearing Audiogram Chart View

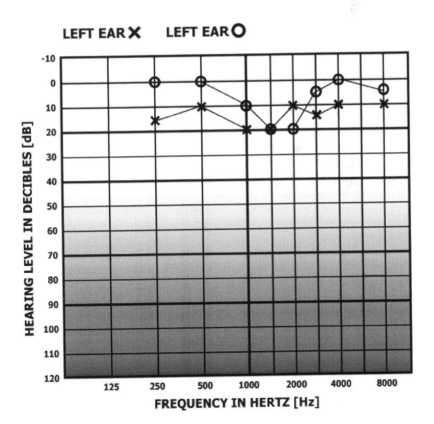

Sensorineural Hearing Loss Audiogram Chart View

LEFT EAR ✕   LEFT EAR ○

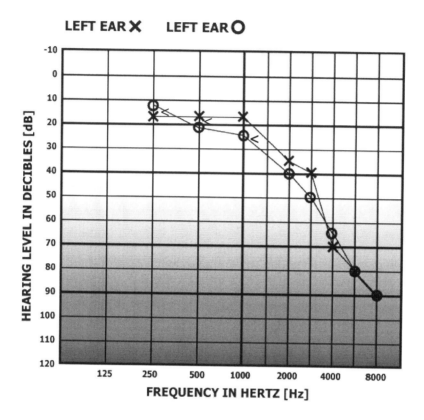

The most common pattern of sensorineural hearing loss is called the "sloping pattern" or a "ski slope pattern." In my practice, over 90% of adults with hearing loss fit this pattern. A sloping hearing loss pattern looks kind of like a ski slope which gradually descends from left to right. In this pattern there is usually normal hearing (less than 25 dB loss) in the lower frequencies and a gradually worsening hearing loss as the frequencies get higher.

A conductive hearing loss is usually caused from problems with earwax (see Section 1), middle ear fluid, or problems with the ossicles, or tympanic membrane. A typical conductive hearing loss pattern is low frequency hearing loss (250 Hz through 1500Hz) up to 60 dB (maximal conductive hearing loss). As an ear surgeon, in many cases of conductive hearing loss, I can often significantly improve hearing with surgical and/or medical treatments.

Conductive Hearing Loss Audiogram Chart View

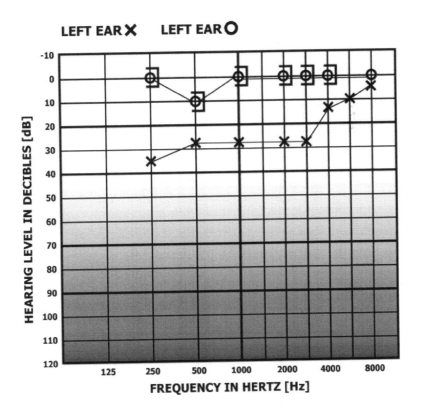

An accurate audiogram is a very important first step to hearing better. An audiogram is critical in determining the type of your hearing loss: conductive, mixed or sensorineural. The test also helps indicate the severity of your hearing loss and by using speech testing, how well you will do with hearing aids

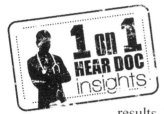

.   When you finally get up the courage to go to a hearing provider's office and get an audiogram, often the provider will hesitate in providing you with a copy of your test results. This practice is illegal. Many hearing aid providers worry that you will take the audiogram results to another hearing provider's office and shop for cheaper hearing aids. You are always entitled to a copy of any personal medical records with few exceptions. The Health Information Portability and Accountability Act (HIPAA) which became Federal law in 1996, entitles you to a copy of your hearing test and most other medical information, although sometimes providers may collect a small fee (usually $15) for copying.

Many hearing aid providers will give you a copy of a very confusing sample audiogram with a large oval drawn in the center called a "speech banana" (see graph on right) and dozens of little pictures on it including alphabet letters, chainsaws, motorcycles, musical notes, and other characters.

Although this form is widely distributed from many hearing aid dispensers' offices, audiologists' offices and some ENT offices, the form has always tended to be confusing.   In my office, I use a simplified form to help patients understand their hearing loss. A copy of your hearing test is the key to obtaining the best hearing aids for your specific hearing loss.

Common "Speech Banana" Audiogram

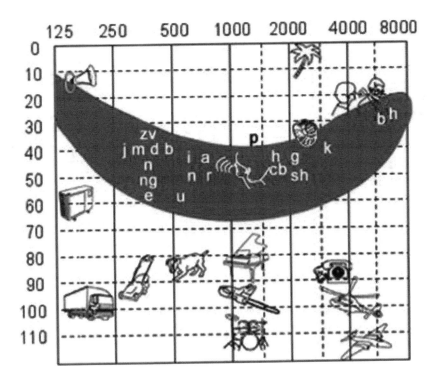

If you have hearing loss, surgery will not correct it and if it does, it will only last for a few years, then you will have to get hearing aids anyway.

FICTION

In about 5-10% of people with hearing loss, it is correctable with medical and/or surgical methods without the use of hearing aids.

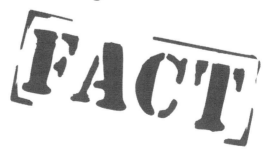

Chapter 9

Restoring Hearing without Hearing Aids

Surgically Correctable Types of Hearing Loss.

As an ear surgeon, when I evaluate a patient for hearing loss, I am always looking to answer the following question: "Can I potentially treat this patient with surgery or medicine to restore hearing?"

I saw a patient for a hearing evaluation many years ago while I was an ENT physician, training in residency. He was an elderly gentleman who came to my clinic because of rapidly progressive hearing loss over the previous year. There were several family members that came with him

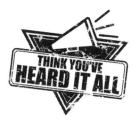

to the appointment. Clearly, they were also very concerned about his hearing. I asked him some simple questions about his hearing and examined him with my surgical microscope. When I looked in the first ear, I immediately noticed something strange. Although he had some ear wax present, it looked very different than normal and oddly it appeared to have fibers within it. I used my forceps to carefully grasp it and gently removed it from the ear canal. It was a small cotton ball! Then I noticed another, and another and another. By the time I was done, I had removed no less than four cotton balls from each ear! His hearing was immediately restored and he was quite elated. His family members called it a "miracle." Afterwards, the patient commented that he had wondered where the cotton ends from his cotton swabs had been disappearing to! It really made me feel great to restore his hearing so quickly and immediately. Unfortunately, hearing restoration is not usually this simple.

There are many other conditions which can cause hearing loss that can be corrected by an ENT doctor such as:

- Simple impacted earwax

- Swelling of the ear canal from infection

- Swelling of the ear canal from boney growths called exostoses (from prolonged cold water exposure, usually seen in surfers and scuba divers)

- Foreign bodies of the ear canal (like cotton swabs, and even insects!)

- Holes (perforations) in the tympanic membrane/middle ear

- Tumors of the ear canal/tympanic membrane

- Missing or misshaped ear bones present at birth or due to injury

- Chronic middle ear or mastoid infections (see below)

Antibiotics have not always been readily available in medical practice in the United States. The first widely available antibiotic was penicillin in 1945. Prior to the introduction of penicillin, ear infections were treated with folk medicine like:

- Blowing hot smoke into the ear canal

- Pouring hot oil into the ear canal

These methods were marginally effective. ENT surgeons developed surgical procedures to remove infection from ears and from mastoid bones behind the ear canal. Since they did not have antibiotics, many early 20th century general practitioners became skilled at "lancing" infected tympanic membranes to release the pressure and infectious material from the middle ear, thereby hoping to resolve ear infections. Many mastoidectomies were also performed in the pre-antibiotic era, which were often life-saving, preventing the spread of infection to deeper structures and the brain, which could result in severe complication and even death. These procedures were initially performed using metal devices with a handle and small cup at the end called "curettes" to scrape out infected bones. As ear surgery modernized and progressed, surgeons started using dental type drills to remove infected mastoid bone to cure ear and mastoid infections.

Mastoid [mas-toid] **Bone**
Located behind and connected to the middle ear consists of air spaces (mastoid cells).

One of my favorite surgical training exercises while in ENT residency was the "Temporal Bone Lab" a.k.a. "T-bone Lab." In the T-bone lab an ENT resident spends many hours practicing removal of mastoid bone from a cadaver ear. I used a surgical microscope and special tiny drills to carefully remove the affected bone and preserve the vital inner ear structures. Since completing my ENT residency, I have examined many patients who were born before the antibiotic era. Often these patients have had severe ear or mastoid infections which have led to scar tissue development of the middle ear structures and subsequent hearing loss. Although their ear infections have been gone for years, some patients are often left with permanent hearing loss which is generally not surgically correctable. The ear and mastoid infections often create microscopic holes (or perforations) in the tympanic membrane. Although tympanic membrane perforations are fairly common in younger patients with a history of chronic ear infections, they are much less common in the elderly.

Another condition which I frequently see is ear canal exostoses. These are benign boney growths of the ear canal which grow in response to repeated exposure to cold water in the ear canals. If you have a past history of chronic cold water exposure from activities such as surfing, scuba diving, swimming in cold mountain streams or other cold water, you may have developed this condition. The boney growths grow very slowly. These growths are very easy for me to diagnose through a simple otoscopic exam. If it is severe, the ear canal can become completely blocked, which can result in hearing loss. Treatment for this condition includes surgical removal of the boney growths, which usually results in restoration of hearing.

Another surgically correctable condition is called otosclerosis, which literally means hardening of the ear bones. Specifically the stapes bone (stirrup bone) becomes fixed in its footplate connection to the inner ear. When it becomes fixed, sound wave energy doesn't transmit well through the bone and this usually results in conductive hearing loss (see Section 1). This condition has a strong hereditary trait and is genetically inherited. For many years ENT physicians treated this condition by simply surgically fracturing the stapes bone to loosen it and restore hearing. This, however, only produced short-lived improvement in hearing which slowly deteriorated again over time.

 Stapes [stey-peez] **Bone**
The smallest of the ossicles which connects to the cochelea.

A surgical procedure was developed to treat this condition which is called stapedectomy. This procedure became more common as microscopes were developed to be used during surgery. When I assisted in my first stapedectomy procedure as a third year medical student, the experience was fascinating to me. I decided at that moment to become an ENT surgeon!

When an ear bone (ossicle) is broken or missing they can often be replaced using a surgical technique called "ossiculoplasty".

Ossicles [os-i-k*uh* l]
The three tiny bones in the middle of the ear that conduct sound energy.

Many different ear bone replacements, which are called "prostheses", have been developed over the years. Hearing restoration using prostheses is generally, but not always, successful. Each year new and improved prostheses are developed to reduce complications and have greater success in hearing restoration. Some of the many problems that can occur after surgery include:

- Infection
- Extrusion or Dislodging of the prosthesis
- Vertigo
- Worsening of hearing loss

Despite the risk of complications, I have many patients who now hear quite well with ossicular prostheses that have been in place for many years.

It was 1988 and I was a third year medical student doing a rotation at the University of Illinois Eye and Ear Hospital in Chicago, Illinois. I was working with attending physician, Dr. Edward Applebaum, a renowned ear surgeon. We had a 34-year-old female patient who had otosclerosis and significant hearing loss in her left ear for many years. Dr. Applebaum performed the surgery with the patient sedated under local anesthesia. He had the operating room lights dimmed and it was completely dark with the notable exception of the piercing light from the high-powered surgical microscope illuminating the ear structures. He had soft classical music playing in the background to create a relaxing, comfortable operating room working environment for the operating room staff members— it was a surreal experience for me. He lifted the tympanic membrane and removed the fixed stapes bone and placed a tiny (4mm long) prosthesis (with 0.8mm diameter piston composed of Teflon coupled to a platinum wire) and placed a patch around the prosthesis. He then replaced the tympanic membrane to its normal position. While still in the operating room, Dr. Applebaum immediately tested the patient's hearing using a sterilized metal tuning fork. The surgery was successful! The patient signaled that she could now hear the tones and her hearing was immediately restored! That day in surgery with Dr. Applebaum made an impact on my professional life. I decided then and there to devote my life to helping people hear!

One of the most common surgical procedures that I perform to restore hearing is called myringotomy. A myringotomy is a procedure in which a tiny opening is created in the tympanic membrane, usually to remove fluid from the middle ear which is causing hearing loss. A special tiny tube is often placed temporarily. It is one of the most common elective surgeries performed in the U.S. today. I most frequently perform myringotomies in my younger pediatric ENT patients but I also sometimes perform this procedure in adults to restore hearing.

Many patients develop hearing loss from chronic middle ear infections which can create persistent fluid in the middle ear, resulting in conductive hearing loss. If the fluid does not resolve with medical treatments such as antibiotic therapy, a myringotomy is sometimes required to restore hearing. The tympanic membrane is tiny—only about 8 mm in diameter. When I perform a myringotomy, I use the surgical microscope and special small instruments to create a hole in the tympanic membrane which on average measures about 3mm in length. Naturally, it is of absolute importance that the patient holds very still during this procedure. Therefore, when this procedure is done on children, general anesthesia in a hospital setting is required. In adults, a myringotomy is a simple, painless 90-second procedure which I perform in my office using one of my surgical microscopes and one drop of anesthesia on the tympanic membrane itself. I don't usually need to perform any painful injections of the ear canal, although I have known some ENT physicians that do. In most cases, hearing is immediately restored after the procedure. I usually have the patient's hearing re-tested post-operatively to recheck their hearing status. Many times after I perform the procedure and remove the middle ear fluid, I insert a 3.0 mm diameter tube to keep the hole open, thereby preventing re-accumulation of the fluid and prolonging hearing restoration. These "ear tubes" usually last about 10 months before falling out, but can last up to 4-5 years, depending on the type of tube which is used.

Conductive hearing loss can also be caused by persistent holes in the eardrum and this situation is usually surgically correctable. These holes can also create a communication between the outside world and the middle ear which may lead to chronic ear infections. These holes are called perforations and result from injury, chronic infection, or can even be from previous ear surgery. Rarely, the skin cells from the ear canal can slowly grow through a perforation and fill the middle ear, destroying the ossicles and creating chronic infection resulting in a condition called cholesteatoma.

 Cholesteatoma [kə-lĕs'tē-ə-tō'mə]
An abnormal growth of skin cells in the middle ear and mastoid.

Perforations can be surgically repaired using several different techniques including patching the hole with fascia (the outer layer of a muscle above the ear—clench your teeth and you can feel it move with your fingers), synthetic materials and other materials.

Occasionally, patients will have profound loss of hearing in both ears. In this situation, whether it is in children or adults, profound hearing loss in both ears means they may not have any useable hearing. Another surgical option is to restore hearing is a cochlear implant. This surgical procedure is reserved for patients who would not receive any benefit from traditional hearing aids. A cochlear implant is a high-tech surgical procedure in which a tiny electrode array is threaded into the inner ear (cochlea) and attached to a micro-computer processing device which looks like a large hearing aid. Sounds are transformed in the device to electrical impulses that directly stimulate the nerve of hearing in the cochlea. The success with this device has been remarkable. Many patients are often able to hear well enough to use the telephone and understand speech without reading lips or any other visual cues.

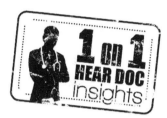

Repair of perforations is successful in over 90% of patients in my practice and frequently, but not always, restore hearing. If cholesteatoma is present in the middle ear and/or mastoid, much more extensive surgical procedures are usually required to remove the disease and attempt to restore hearing. It is important to note in patients with cholesteatoma, the goal of surgery is usually not to restore hearing as much as to provide the patient with a safe, infection-free ear.

Since I have a passion for surgical restoration of hearing, when I examine patients I am always looking for conditions such as:

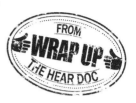

- Tympanic membrane perforations
- Middle ear fluid accumulation
- Correctable blockage of the ear canals
- Otosclerosis
- Cholesteatoma
- Other surgically correctable types of hearing loss

Unfortunately, only about 5-10% of patients that I examine with hearing loss have any of these conditions that can be helped with surgical procedures. The remaining 90% of patients need hearing aids to restore their hearing

....

"It takes five years to learn how to operate and twenty years to learn when not to."

-Anonymous

....

"My Hearing loss cannot be helped."

FICTION

Hearing aids are effective in restoring hearing in over 90% of my adult patients. You just have to summon the courage to do something. Hearing loss is treatable.

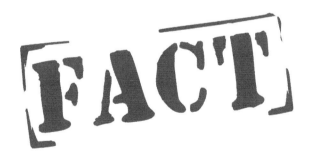

SECTION 3
The Hearing Aid (The Device)

This section is the heart of this book. The passion behind writing this book was born out of sharing the following information about hearing aids that is summed up in the fact statement on the corresponding page of this spread.

The following topics will be covered in this section:

- The Hearing Aid
- Why Are Hearing Aids So Expensive?
- The Secrets to Buying a Hearing Aid
- Troubleshooting your Hearing Aids

Hearing aids always have problems with feedback and squealing noises.

FICTION

Today's hearing aids are sophisticated devices. They have digital noise control features, dual microphones and receiver-in-the-canal technology which help to eliminate feedback noise and create a comfortable hearing experience.

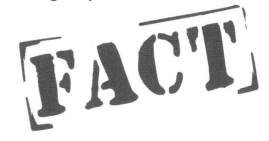

Chapter 10
The Hearing Aid

If you've read the first two sections of this book, you now know a lot about hearing loss, ear anatomy and common surgical procedures of the ear. You also probably have a pretty good idea whether or not you have hearing loss. That could even be why you picked up this book in the first place. Hopefully you now understand more about the remarkably complex structure of the human ear. As I mentioned earlier in the book, 90-95% of the patients that I see in my ENT clinic do not have a surgically correctable hearing loss condition. Therefore, if you are reading this book and you believe that you have hearing loss, there is at least a 90% chance that hearing aids are needed to correct your hearing loss.

 Decibels [des-*uh*-bel, -b*uh* l]
A measure of sound intensity (loudness).

Now it's time for a little history lesson. The first "aid to hearing" was not a device at all but simply a cupped hand. Try it. Have someone speak to you from across the room and listen to the person's voice both with and without your hand cupped behind one of your ears. It is estimated that the sound is amplified about 4 or 5 dB (Decibels). Although this is only a mild increase, it does help some people hear better and this form of amplification focuses your hearing to the speaker, partially blocking out the other sounds around you. With this in mind, early pioneers developed hearing aid "horns" or "ear trumpets," huge devices which were connected with a funnel into the ear canal. Of course, today those horns are a joke and no one uses them, although some of you reading this book may have had a granddad that used one many years ago.

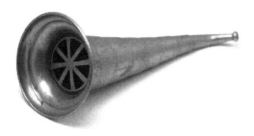

The ear trumpets were in use well into the 20th century, until batteries and wearable hearing aids were developed.

Probably, more than anything else, the first innovation which revolutionized hearing restoration was battery development. The first hearing aids were worn on your body and were called "body aids." They were quite large, mostly due to the size of the battery and the circuitry. The first electronic hearing aid was called the Akouphone and was developed in 1898 by Miller Reese Hutchinson. It was created with a carbon transmitter to be portable. It was quite large and fit into purses or other accessories. I imagine those were about as big as the old cellular telephones called "bag phones." Remember those?

In 1913 the Siemens Company designed an electronic amplifying hearing aid. It was large and bulky, about the size of a "tall cigar box," and was not easily portable. It had a speaker that fit into the ear.

By the 1930's hearing aids had become much smaller and lighter with the development of vacuum tube technology and smaller batteries. It was at this point that hearing aids became somewhat more popular with the public. Transistors and integrated circuits lead to further miniaturization of hearing aids and even greater acceptance.

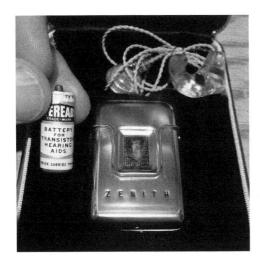

Zenith was the first company to offer "all-transistor" hearing aids in 1952, called the Microtone Transimatic.

The end of the transistor hearing aid was marked by the creation of the integrated circuit by Jack Kilby at Texas Instruments in 1958. By far the greatest development in the history of hearing aids, second only to battery and circuitry miniaturization, was the development of fully digital hearing aids. The first digital hearing aids were actually a hybrid of analog and digital technologies. The first commercial digital hearing aid was created in 1987 by the Nicolet Corporation. In addition to the Nicolet Corporation, Bell Laboratories expanded upon the hearing aid business by developing a hybrid analog-digital hearing aid. Even though early research on this hearing aid was successful, AT&T, the parent company of Bell Laboratories, pulled out of the hearing aid market and sold its rights to Resound Corporation in 1987. When the digital hearing aid was put on the market, it was instantaneously successful. This development marked the beginning of major changes to the hearing aid and the hearing aid industry.

Today, most hearing aids are fully digitalized. I rarely recommend the older technology analog hearing aids anymore, so I will focus my discussion here on digital hearing aids. Digital hearing aids are tiny, amazing devices. They make soft sounds louder and loud sounds softer and they are physically and acoustically very comfortable to wear. Some of the many other benefits of digital hearing aids include:

- Automatic Volume Control
- Digital Feedback (squealing) Reduction
- Digital Noise Reduction
- Digital Speech Enhancement
- Digital Background Noise Reduction
- Hearing Aid to Hearing Aid (ear-to-ear) Communication
- Digital Tinnitus Reduction

OK, end of history lesson...

After you have visited a hearing a professional, your hearing health history has been reviewed, your ears have been carefully examined, and a diagnostic audiogram has been performed, you will have a pretty good idea of your overall hearing status. You should receive the following information:

- The type of your hearing loss (conductive vs. sensorineural vs. mixed).

- The severity of your hearing loss.

- Your speech discrimination (understanding) ability.

- Existing medical ear conditions or deformities.

All of these factors are taken into consideration when selecting the most appropriate hearing aids for you. The information is used by the hearing professional to determine the type of hearing aid which will be best suited for you and your hearing aid amplification "prescription." It is this prescription that is programmed directly into your new digital hearing aids, using a programming computer. The programming procedure results in hearing aids that are specifically customized for you and fit only you and your actual hearing loss pattern. This results in maximum sound comfort and understanding of speech.

The basic components of a digital hearing aid

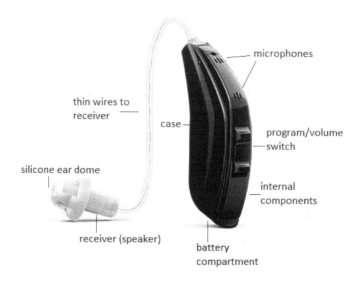

- Microphone(s)

- Analog to Digital Converter

- Digital Sound Processor/Amplifier

- Digital to Analog Converter

- Receiver (speaker)

- Volume control (usually automatically controlled)

- Battery

- On/Off switch

- Telecoil

- Hearing Aid Case

- Bluetooth Transmitter

The first major component of a hearing aid is the **microphone**, which picks up sounds in your environment and converts them into electrical signals. Microphone input is converted to digital signals that are processed and shaped. Many hearing aids now have two microphones. The microphones are usually lined up horizontally and spaced at least 8 millimeters (mm) apart, so that the microphone in the front picks up sounds that originate in front of you a split second before the microphone in the rear. The sound processor uses this information to "focus" on the sound, which in most cases is the speaker's voice (who is in front of you) and the processor ignores the sounds which are coming from behind you (background noises). Obviously this doesn't work as well when both the speaker's voice and the noise are coming from the same direction (like when someone is calling your name behind you in a soft voice). Another microphone technology is directional microphones that capture sound from a specific direction, which is usually from in front of you. These microphone signals are also shaped by the digital sound processor.

The hearing aid **analog to digital converter** takes microphone input and converts it to digital signals which are altered and shaped by the **digital sound processor (DSP).** The DSP is the control center of a digital hearing aid. It is a tiny computer chip inside of every digital hearing aid. It increases the intensity of the signals from the microphone, filters out unwanted sounds, and modifies the sounds based on prescribed programs. These programs can easily be changed in many different ways to provide optimal sound comfort and speech understanding for you. Only sounds which are important to your understanding of speech are amplified. Other sounds such as background noise, loud noises, and circuit noise are suppressed based on your customized program.

The fourth component of a hearing aid is the **digital to analog converter.** It converts the specially processed digital signal back into an analog signal which is amplified and can then be perceived as sound. It's worth noting that we cannot hear digital signals, therefore the digital signals must be converted back to analog signals which are amplified and heard by our ears.

The **receiver** is the speaker of the hearing aid. It produces the sound waves which are heard. The receiver is sometimes located within the case of the hearing aid and in some designs it is located within the ear canal itself, connected to the hearing aid by wires.

Many experienced hearing aid wearers like to have a **volume control**, which is usually a small button which can be rotated with one finger either forward (to increase volume) or backwards (to decrease volume). However, modern hearing aid volume levels are adjusted automatically in the digital sound processor (DSP) and there is usually no need for a volume control. If a patient is accustomed to having a volume control, it can easily be added to a hearing aid and digitally programmed to increase or decrease the receiver output. I usually discourage adding volume control knobs anymore, as the processors these days are sophisticated and control volume automatically.

The hearing aid **battery** is the energy source which provides power for modern hearing aids. The most common type of battery used is the zinc-air battery. Many different battery sizes are available based on how much power is needed to run the hearing aid and the size of battery that will actually fit inside the hearing aid case.

Here are the four most common battery sizes:

- 10   Size (5.8 mm x 3.6 mm).

- 13   Size (7.9 mm x 5.4 mm)

- 312   Size (7.9 mm x 3.6 mm)

- 675   Size (11.6 mm x 5.4 mm)

The #10 battery is very small and has a diameter of only 5.8 mm which is about the length of a small grain of rice. The 675 battery is 11.6 mm in diameter which is about the size of a green pea.

I almost always recommend that hearing aids have a **telecoil**. This is a simple copper coil device which allows use of a standard telephone and some cellular phones with the hearing aid. When the hearing aid senses the telephone receiver is in close proximity, it automatically switches to the telecoil instead of the microphone to pick up sound. This virtually eliminates feedback and provides for improved sound quality. Some hearing aids require you to flip a switch, usually marked with a "T" to turn on the telecoil, but I recommend an automatic built in switch.

Telecoils are also used for **looped hearing systems**. In many public places such as auditoriums and movie theatres, the sound is broadcast using a magnetic loop which can be picked up by a standard hearing aid telecoil directly into hearing aids. In some foreign countries such as Denmark, there is extensive use of looped hearing systems in almost all public places. The telecoil is an inexpensive option which is available in all but the tiniest hearing aids.

The hearing aid **on and off switch** simply does what it says. When the hearing aids are out of the ear they should be switched off to save the battery and prevent feedback noise. A simple way to turn off a hearing aid is to open the battery compartment door. This action not only turns the hearing aid off, it also allows the hearing aid circuitry to dry out when not in use.

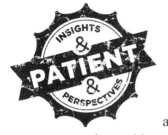

Some companies have developed rechargeable hearing aid batteries. These batteries are more expensive, but some of my patients like them. Most patients choose disposable batteries which cost about $1 US per cell and usually last 7-10 days with normal wear. I like to sell hearing aid batteries in my office which are shipped directly to me from the battery manufacturers. This way I know my patients are obtaining fresh, powerful hearing aid batteries which have not been sitting in a hot warehouse for months before they were purchased. In my experience, most hearing aid batteries last about the same amount of time, regardless of the manufacturer, as long as they are fresh. Since they are very small (particularly sizes 10 and 312), some battery companies package them with an elongated pull tab which help you to place them into the hearing aid, if you have manual dexterity problems. (For example, arthritis.)

One of the factors which reduce the lifespan of a hearing aid more than anything else is moisture. I usually recommend that my patients remove their hearing aids at night and turn them off by opening the battery door. I also recommend hearing aid drying devices which I provide my patients for a nominal fee. These devices can significantly prolong the life of a hearing aid—by years! Recently, several different hearing aid manufacturers have also developed moisture resistant hearing aids, in which the internal components are plasma-coated at the molecular level to repel the effects of moisture.

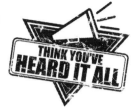

I had one particular hearing aid patient who purchased a new, high quality, behind-the-ear hearing aids from my office and three days later he returned to the office saying that they no longer worked! I performed a check of the hearing aids and both were dead with corrosion in the battery compartment. I returned them to the factory for replacement and the new hearing aids were fit a few days later. After another three days the patient again returned stating that the replacements were also dead! I returned both hearing aids to the factory and ordered hearing aids from another manufacturer. The same thing happened with the other maker's aids. By this time both the patient and I were getting very frustrated. I examined the battery compartment of the 4th set of replacement aids with my surgical microscope and once again the battery contacts were corroded and green with only 3 days of use. I asked the patient if he had gotten them wet or accidently stepped in the shower with them and he replied "No." I asked him what kind of work he did and he said he worked outdoors as a farmer. I determined that his sweat was of a particular composition that caused corrosion of the battery compartment when it leaked in. I solved the problem by ordering a type of hearing aid which had a waterproof seal on the battery compartment door which did not allow any moisture in at all. He was fit with these hearing aids and subsequently did quite well.

The **hearing aid case** holds all the components together. It is the "chassis" of the hearing aid. It is usually made of a durable plastic. For the "behind-the-ear" type of hearing aids, the case has a standard design and shape based on the manufacturer's preference. For custom fitted "in-the-ear" type of hearing aids, the case is custom made at the factory based on an impression (mold) of your ear. Obtaining an ear impression is a simple process in which I first place cotton or a foam plug in the ear canal attached to a string. I then use a two-part silicone material which is gently injected into your ear canal and allowed to harden in about 4-5 minutes. It is removed along with the cotton/foam and an exact mold of the ear canal is made. The impression is either mailed to the hearing aid factory or placed in a 3-D scanning device and sent to the factory electronically to make a custom hearing aid.

For many years hearing aid cases came in only one color–beige. Fortunately, this trend is reversing. A huge palate of colors are now available to customize hearing aid cases, including grey, black, brown, silver, and also exotic colors like leopard print, hot pink and even clear plastic cases. I believe that with increased acceptance of devices worn on the ear, such as Bluetooth devices for cell phones and ear buds for iPods, more and more patients will want to make a statement with their hearing aids to show others that they are confident and want to hear well.

Finally, many modern hearing aids have built-in **Bluetooth®** **technology**. Bluetooth is short range wireless radiofrequency which allows connectivity between other Bluetooth devices (or Bluetooth compatible devices). I highly recommend this technology be included in a hearing aid when your budget allows. Bluetooth (and other transmission frequencies) make hearing aid programming easier and allow hearing aids to "talk" to each other and coordinate for better speech understanding, volume control and directionality of sound. Remote control devices can also be easily paired to hearing aids with radio frequency, enabling you to easily change between programs, particularly if you have manual dexterity problems.

Bluetooth allows wireless streaming of a variety of technology devices including:

- Television
- Telephone
- Cellular phones
- Digital music players
- Computers

Think this is what a hearing aid looks like?

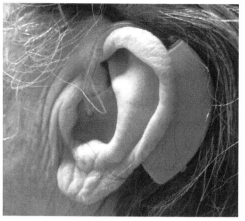

If so, think again...

Hearing aids come in many different styles. Some are selected based on patient preference, while other styles are chosen by the hearing aid dispenser based on the patient's hearing loss for maximum benefit.

There are six basic styles of hearing aids:

- **B**ehind **T**he **E**ar (**BTE**)
- Mini **B**ehind **T**he **E**ar (**Mini BTE**---AKA *On The Ear* - **OTE**)
- **R**eceiver **I**n the ear **C**anal (**RIC**---AKA - **RITE**)

Custom Molded Hearing Aids:

- **I**n **T**he **E**ar (**ITE**)
- **I**n **T**he **C**anal (**ITC**)
- **C**ompletely **I**n the ear **C**anal (**CIC**)

Images provided by

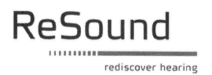

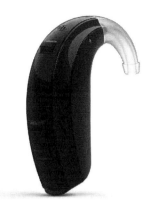

Behind The Ear (BTE)

Plastic tubing carries sound to a soft silicone ear dome or a custom ear mold (not shown).

Benefits: Larger size makes it easier to manipulate. It can be used to fit almost all types of hearing loss. It is excellent for severe or profound hearing losses. BTE devices can accommodate a larger battery (up to size 675--- which may last longer).

They can also accommodate two microphones and a manual volume control (if desired).

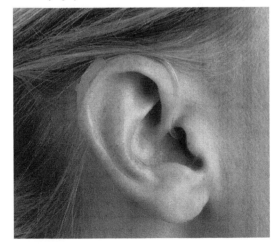

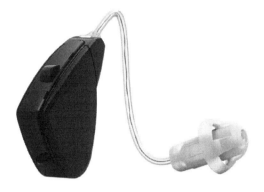

Mini behind the ear (Mini BTE)

Plastic tube connects to a soft silicone earbud in the ear canal.

Benefits: Leaves the ear canal open for more natural sound, especially your own voice. No custom mold required, but can be used. It can accommodate two microphones. It can also have a manual volume control.

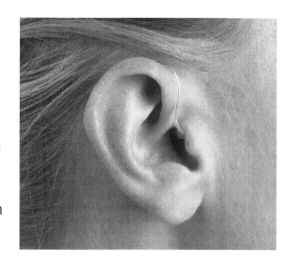

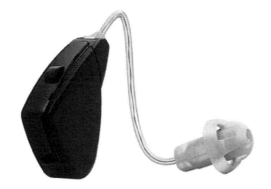

Receiver in canal (RIC)

Microphone and digital processor are behind the ear; connected with tiny wires to a receiver in an earbud or custom mold in the canal.

Benefits: One of the most cosmetically pleasing devices. It can provide superior sound quality. It is the most common type of hearing aid dispensed by Dr. Frantz.

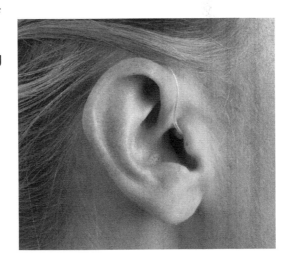

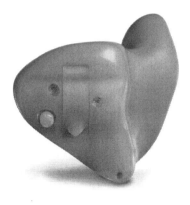

In the ear (ITE)

Custom-made device which fits in the outer ear.

Benefits: Easy to insert; can have a directional microphone or two microphones and volume control; easy to use with the telephone. It is a good choice for low frequency hearing losses. It may produce an occlusion effect (may feel "plugged up").

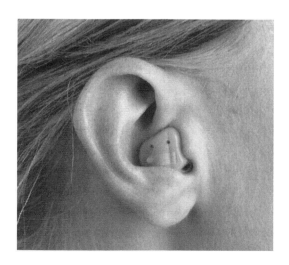

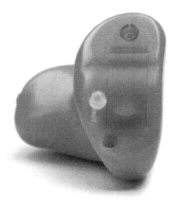

In the canal (ITC)

Custom-made device which fits into the ear canal opening.

Benefits: Good cosmetic appearance; large enough for two microphones and volume control. It is also a good choice for low frequency hearing losses. It may also produce an occlusion effect.

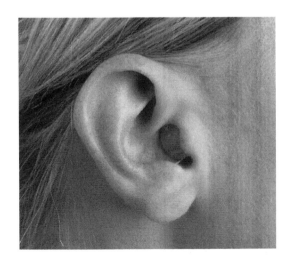

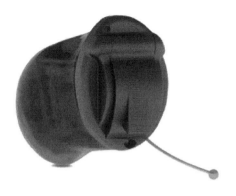

Completely in the canal (CIC)

Fits entirely in the ear canal. Inserted and removed by an insertion handle.

Benefits: Excellent cosmetic appearance; least visible; easy to use with telephone. Can only accommodate one microphone. Must use the smallest battery size (10). May produce occlusion.

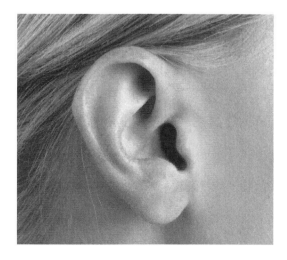

I often see patients who have profound loss in one ear which is unaidable (a "dead" ear) with useable hearing in the opposite (contralateral) ear. These patients suffer from a profound hearing loss in one ear for various reasons. They usually present to 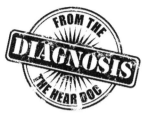 my office thinking that they will never have any hearing in the profoundly deaf ear and tell me about problems with conversations, especially when the speech is located towards the deaf ear. Regardless of whether the opposite (hearing) ear has normal hearing or some degree of hearing loss, there is a solution. In the past, the CROS hearing aids required a bulky pair of eyeglasses which contained a wire through the frame to connect the ears, or slim wires which connected the right and left hearing aids behind the neck, today those are considered "vintage" and are only of interest for collectors.

There is a seventh type of hearing aids called a CROS (**C**ontralateral **R**outing **O**f the **S**ignal). These are used for patients with only one hearing ear. This is a highly sophisticated hearing aid system requiring two hearing aids, one of which in placed in the deaf ear and the other is placed in the hearing ear. The hearing aid in the deaf ear consists of only a microphone and transmission system. The signals are sent to the better hearing ear's hearing aid via Bluetooth or other transmission system. CROS hearing aids make it possible for patients to hear sounds from the deaf ear side in the good (opposite side) ear. The overall acceptance of CROS hearing aid systems versus wearing only one hearing aid (in the hearing ear) in my practice is excellent, however many individuals with unilateral deafness prefer to use only one hearing aid in the better ear.

All hearing aids are expensive and all hearing professionals have a preferred manufacturer from which they get their hearing aids, because they are so expensive to make.

FICTION

Buying hearing aids is a bullet-proof experience, you can test-drive different ones—until you find the brand, manufacturer and style that have the right features for you and are within your budget.

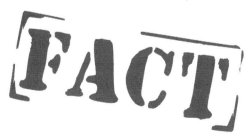

Chapter 11

Why Are Hearing Aids so Expensive?

So why are hearing aids so expensive? That's a good question. One of the most common reasons people who need hearing aids don't get them is because of the high cost. I think I've found a solution that will benefit many people, but first I'll give you a little history of pricing that will help you understand how things are done. So bear with me, I'll describe my solution in a few pages – and eventually, I will even give you some ideas on how to get a hearing aid at a reduced cost or possibly even for free.

When I first began dispensing hearing aids in my practice in 1994, the average price of a hearing aid was $670. Digital hearing aids became more popular in 1995 and with the advent of the CIC hearing aid, the average cost of a digital hearing aid jumped to $910. Since 1995, the average retail cost of a hearing aid has increased above the rate of inflation with each new technological advance. As of 2012, the average retail price for a pair of high-quality digital hearing aids, nationwide, jumped to $4,200.

There are currently about 22 major hearing aid manufacturers and each has dozens of different models. These instruments all have amazing technology and are all proven to help you hear, but they are certainly very expensive. Is the high price of hearing aids due to expensive production costs? The actual cost to produce a hearing aid is difficult to determine from the hearing aid manufacturers. Six major manufacturers provide hearing aids to the US Veteran's Administration.

Lucille Beck, Director, Audiology and Speech Pathology Service - Veterans Affairs, reported in 2011 that the VA dispensed 561,212 hearing aids in 2010, about 20% of **all** hearing aids dispensed in the U.S. that year. The average manufacturer cost of a hearing aid to the VA was $348.15.

How much does a private practice pay for hearing aids that they dispense? Typically, they buy either direct from the manufacturer or from a "buying group," in order to reduce costs. The buying groups negotiate lower prices from manufacturers based on volume sold and resell premium hearing aids to private practices for an average wholesale cost of $900 to $1,850 each.

The private practice's average wholesale cost of a hearing aid is currently approximately $1,200 each ($2,400 per pair) and the average retail selling price is about $4,200 per pair. This equates to over a 500 percent markup from the estimated manufacturer production cost ($800 or less per pair) to retail ($4,200 per pair) for two hearing aids! A *2009 Consumer Reports* survey noted that there is an average retail markup of 117 percent over wholesale cost by hearing aid dispensers in the US.

The high cost of hearing aids is therefore NOT due to production costs. The high cost of hearing aids is due to the combination of an average $750 markup from the manufacturer and a $1,200 - $2,000 retail markup by the hearing professional. Is the high retail markup of hearing aids due to the time spent in fitting/dispensing them? The average number of patient visits to properly test hearing and fit hearing aids is about 3 office visits of approximately one hour duration each.

The audiologist typically spends an additional 1 hour for the hearing exam (audiogram) and initial consultation, so they typically spend a total of about 4 hours per hearing aid fitting per patient.

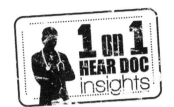

When I turned 43-years-old a few years ago, I began to notice that while I was performing certain surgical procedures, I could not clearly see some of the anatomical structures, such as arteries and nerves. I knew that I had probably gradually developed a case of presbyopia (eye-site of advancing age). At the time I didn't go to my eye doctor and have my eyes tested. Instead I simply went to my local pharmacy and bought a $12 pair of reading glasses. The difference was immediate and striking. When I began wearing my new reading glasses in the operating room, surgical structures became clear and sharp. Unfortunately this is not the case for hearing restoration. If you're considering purchasing a pair of high quality, custom fitted digital hearing aids from a hearing professional such as an ENT or audiologist, you can expect to pay $4,000 to $7,000. To make matters worse, hearing aids are generally not covered by most insurance plans or Medicare, so the cost is usually all out of pocket.

Most hearing aid dispensers typically include unlimited free office visits for adjustment, repair and routine hearing aid service during the trial period (usually 30-45 days) and sometimes for the lifetime of the hearing aid. All of these office visits and personnel costs are typically bundled into the initial price of the hearing aids resulting in higher retail prices.

It's a frustrating dilemma. Why have digital improvements helped us develop cheaper smart phones, flat screen TVs, laptop computers, and tablets. Yet the same kind of technological advancements have only caused the price of hearing aids to increase—typically, impacting a retired population on fixed incomes! In my research for this book, I came across an interesting comparison which looked at the production costs/profit margins for an Apple iPad versus a hearing aid called, "Why Does a Hearing Aid Cost Six Times more than an iPad?" Below is that cost breakdown comparison. It was written based on (1) an article in the *Economist* magazine discussing the cost breakdown of making and distributing an iPad, (2) a German government article discussing (in English, fortunately) the cost breakdown and profits of Phonak and other hearing aid manufacturers required as part of a merger request. This paper first appeared in a blog hosted by Patrick Freuler. It was written by Ed Belcher and Patrick Freuler. The authors perform a detailed cost structure analysis of both an Apple iPad and a premium hearing aid. In their comparison, they found that although the actual production costs for each device is similar, this accounts for only 8% of a hearing aids retail cost (production + R&D + marketing + overhead + retail markup) versus 55% of an Apple iPad's retail cost. The huge difference in retail price (approximately $500 for an Apple iPad versus $3000 for a premium hearing aid) is mainly due to the retail markup of 15% versus 67% respectively.

Certainly the market for Apple iPads is exponentially larger than that for hearing aids. In 2013 Apple sold an estimated 170 million iPads versus in 2012 only an estimated 10.8 million hearing aids worldwide from all major manufacturers combined.

So, the answer to the question "Why are Hearing Aids so expensive?" is mainly due to the tremendous markup at both the wholesale and retail levels. Unfortunately, the current nationwide push amongst most hearing professionals in the U.S. is for hearing aid "price preservation" to maintain high retail pricing.

The U.S. market penetration for hearing aids is only 20-25% in those who need them; therefore, each retailer only sells a fraction of the potential number of hearing aids which could be sold. If most of the people who needed hearing aids actually bought them, the cost structure would be different. Furthermore, of the 20-25% of people who do purchase hearing aids, (despite the high prices) most of these individuals cannot function without them and would have to live with severe hearing disabilities if they did not purchase – this means that, frankly, they could not function well without them and are forced to buy—regardless of price. So what does that mean for those individuals with mild or moderate hearing loss? Although they need hearing aids, they typically put off the purchase an average of 7- 8 years from when they first notice a hearing problem until the degree of hearing loss worsens.

The average age of patients who purchase hearings aids in my clinic is 71, although the majority of people with hearing loss (65%) are younger than 65.

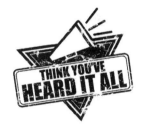

Hearing professionals nationwide have different discount structures from the manufacturers and buying networks based on several factors. In the late 1990's my practice committed to selling a single company's brand of hearing aids for a full year. We were rewarded handsomely for our commitment. We received a significant discount on all our hearing aids (which benefited the bottom line) and we also received an all-expenses paid, first-class tour of Paris and Monte Carlo. Hearing aid companies justify these trips as a cost of doing business to incentivize their sales people (audiologists, physicians, and hearing aid dispensers). Of course, someone must pay for these expensive trips, the costs of which are added to the wholesale cost of the hearing aids.

In 2009 the U.S. pharmaceutical industry began self-regulating gifts to healthcare providers. In an effort to reduce the escalating costs of pharmaceuticals, 54 pharmaceutical companies adopted the PhRMA Code of 2009 which is not law, but a voluntary agreement including many restrictions on marketing to healthcare providers. Some of these restrictions include bans on free, extravagant meals that do not come with an educational value. Non-educational gifts (branded pens, sticky note pads, clipboards) and taking healthcare providers to recreational events were also banned. Educational gifts are allowable, as long as the price does not exceed $100. The PhRMA code also asks that any healthcare provider who acts as a consultant disclose the financial relationship.

So you might be asking, "Should there be federal laws concerning promotional gifts and recreational events given to hearing aid dispensers and audiologists to help reduce hearing aid prices?" Currently, I am not aware of any efforts within the hearing aid industry to create a voluntary agreement to address this issue.

Another reason that hearing aid prices continue to rise is with the marketing of "new" innovations. It seems like every two or three months one or another hearing aid manufacturer comes out with something "new". In reality, most of these "must have" evolutions are simply minor changes in the DSP (microchip) of their "new" and "improved" hearing aid model. The manufacturers typically host a "launch party" for a weekend away in a fun location and invite their loyal dispensers to attend, all expenses paid. During the lavish dinners a flashy presentation is given to communicate the "new innovation" in a very professional and well-presented manner. This announcement is frequently coupled with a special "launch offer" for the new product, such as "Buy 3 new hearing aids and get the 4th free" or "Buy 4 hearing aids and get the new fitting kit for free." The weekend conferences end up having the intended results. When my audiologists attend, they usually return to the practice and counsel patients to buy the new (more expensive) technology, even though last quarter's technology worked very well for our patients. It is my personal opinion that this marketing strategy contributes to further increase hearing aid costs to the consumer, and I'll put my money where my mouth is and be the first to admit that my practice is guilty of this as well. I believe that nationwide, many hearing professionals are convinced that they need to sell a somewhat improved hearing aid in a shiny new shell at increasing prices each year, despite nominal technological advantages.

Something has to be done to make hearing aids more affordable for the people who need them. That is why I am exposing this fact and lifting the veil. While doing research for this book, I determined that my own practice was guilty of most of the cost markups which make hearing aids unaffordable to many of the people who really need them. Although I started dispensing hearing aids in 1995 as an add-on service to my ENT practice, they had become a major profit center, generating approximately 37% of our revenues year over year. I spoke to the staff audiologists about the problems that I found with the high cost of hearing aids and I discovered that they were well aware of this trend (they are compensated by commission based on monthly hearing aid sales). I proposed that we re-structure our practice's hearing aid pricing to make it much more transparent for the end consumer, effectively "unbundling" all of the hearing aid charges. We decided to call the new affordable pricing the "Fee for Service" plan. We started charging only a nominal "fitting fee" per hearing aid plus our actual wholesale cost for the hearing aid. We also started including all office visits within the 30 day trial period at no additional charge. After the 30-day trial is completed, subsequent office visits have a reasonable charge of a $40-$60 per visit, which we refer to as a "co-pay."

So what were the results of this change in our business process and pricing formula? We were able to drastically lower our hearing aid retail prices (by some 25-30%) and this resulted in both a significant increase in sales and much happier patients! My staff audiologists were delighted! Of course, this equated to much less revenue per patient, but the audiologists were quite altruistic and very excited to help many more people hear better, through our new pricing structure.

It is worth noting that we continue to offer our "Worry Free" hearing aid purchase option which has higher upfront costs, but includes free office visits, hearing aid programming and "clean and checks" for a 2-3 year period from the day of purchase. To our surprise, about 20% of our patients still prefer purchasing their hearing aids in this way, despite the significantly higher associated costs.

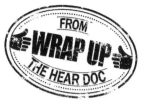

There are a handful of hearing aid dispensers and audiologists in the country who have adopted straight-forward, affordable, "unbundled" hearing aid pricing, as we have done. It is my belief that if this were done on a larger scale, by more ENTs, audiologists, and dispensers nationwide, it would enable many more people to obtain their needed hearing aids. It would also allow current hearing aid wearers to more easily upgrade to new hearing aids when significant advances in technology arise, rather than keeping their current hearing aids for as many years as possible due to the high cost of obtaining new ones. Unfortunately, the current push in the industry amongst hearing aid providers is for hearing aid "price preservation." Sadly, from my perspective, most providers are quite content to keep hearing aid retail prices inflated for maximum profit, even though this pushes away—due to the high costs—about 75% of those who need help with their hearing.

"Hearing aids are expensive and cost about the same, regardless of where you buy them. There are not any programs available to get free or low-cost hearing aids. Once you buy them you are stuck with them, even if they don't help you hear better."

FICTION

Before you purchase hearing aids, know who you are going to visit (ENT vs. audiologist vs. dispenser), know what you want from your new hearing aids before your appointment, bring your spouse or a close friend to the appointment, and avoid "hard sell" pressure sales techniques.

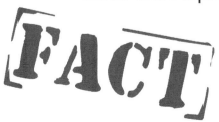

Chapter 12
The Secrets to Buying Hearing Aids

Having read this far, you know that hearing aids are digital, technological marvels which not only improve your hearing but can significantly improve your overall well-being, communication ability, and relationships. Unfortunately, you also have learned that hearing aids are quite expensive at the retail level, making entry into the world of better hearing financially difficult, if not impossible, for many individuals with hearing loss. To make matters even worse, the process of buying a hearing aid can be as confusing as buying a new car! I often see pictures in hearing aid advertisements comparing the size of a small (CIC) hearing aid to a picture of a U.S. dime. There are also advertisements with pricing offers which can be confusing such as:

- **50% OFF – M.S.R.P.!**
- **Buy One Hearing Aid, Get One FREE!**

The ads send confusing or even misleading messages. Get ready because this is the chapter where I will tell you some secrets I have learned, that hopefully you can use to obtain hearing aids at a fair price (and in some cases for free).

The hearing aid industry had little regulation until 1977 when they became class III medical devices (most are now class I or II devices) regulated by the F.D.A. Prior to this time, hearing aids were primarily used as personal amplifiers that could be placed directly into the people's ears. As a result of consumer pressure from Ralph Nader's *Public Citizen* and other senior citizen groups regarding hearing aid sales abuse and consumer fleecing, the FDA decided to regulate the industry.

All 50 states now require a licensed professional to sell hearing aids. In many states there are several types of professionals, with widely varied training, who can legally sell you a hearing aid. Hearing aid dispensers (a sales person) must be licensed in all 50 states. However, the devil is in the details and the training and experience of each individual can vary widely.

As I mentioned earlier, unfortunately, due to expense, only about 25% of people with hearing loss (who really need hearing aids) actually purchase and wear them. That means 75% of those with hearing loss live with a hearing disability. When I examine a patient and find that he/she needs hearing aids, they usually decide to have a second consultation with the office audiologist. If patients decide not to try hearing aids at that time, I have found that on average, they will put off doing something about their hearing for another 18 months before seeking another hearing loss consultation. Practically speaking, for a year and a half that person will miss out on things like: important conversations, interactions, music, and children's voices. In other words, they will not fully experience life's activities due to the untreated hearing disability! Don't let yourself become one of those statistics.

My purpose in writing this book is to enrich the quality of life by helping as many people as possible hear better, each day, in many different circumstances, and in all aspects of their lives. That is also my goal as an ENT physician, and why I got into the profession in the first place. Sometimes better hearing requires a simple office procedure, medication, or maybe even complex microsurgery, but for most people it requires only the acceptance of hearing aids. Patients often ask me if they "need" hearing aids or if I am simply "recommending" them? My question back is, "When do you 'need' to hear?" The answer to this question is simple. When you stop doing certain activities that you used to enjoy or discontinue relationships because of your hearing loss, hearing aids are *needed*. If your hearing loss is not corrected at that point, you will begin withdrawing from life's activities and studies have shown a high likelihood that you will become depressed, which can lead to late life dementia.

Here is my stance - don't withdraw from life and get depressed. Keep active in your relationships, sports, business meetings, family events, social events, religious activities, and stay mentally sharp by simply getting some hearing aids if/when you need them.

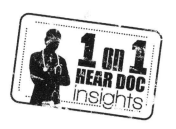

In this chapter, I tell you some secrets to buying hearing aids. I debated how much "insider" information to include in this chapter. When I told one of my regional hearing aid company representatives about writing this book and my chapter on "Secrets to Buying a Hearing Aid," he recommended that I wait until my retirement from practice to publish this book! He echoed my thoughts about the nationwide push for hearing aid price preservation and warned me that I would not be very popular amongst the nation's hearing aid dispensers when this book was published. Well, I'm going to put myself out there and tell you everything I know about how to get hearing aids and start hearing better!

Probably the best kept secret in getting hearing aids is how to get them for free!

You may be surprised to learn that there are many programs available which provide free hearing aids for patients who qualify. The largest and best is the Veterans Administration. The V.A. Health system dispenses about 500,000 free hearing aids to qualified veterans each year.

If you are a qualified veteran with documented service connected hearing loss or even non-service connected hearing loss, you may qualify for this program. There are many circumstances which may qualify you for free hearing aids and audiology services. *The following content is verbatim from the V.A. site:*

"Ensuring access to audiology and eye care services including preventive health (care) services and routine vision testing for all enrolled veterans and those veterans exempt from enrollment. Eyeglasses and **hearing aids must be provided** to the following veterans:

(a) Those with any compensable service-connected disability.

(b) Those who are former Prisoners of War (POWs).

(c) Those who were awarded a Purple Heart.

(d) Those in receipt of benefits under Title 38 United States Code (U.S.C.) 1151.

(e) Those in receipt of an increased pension based on being permanently housebound and in need of regular aid and attendance.

(f) Those with vision or hearing impairment resulting from diseases or the existence of another medical condition for which the veteran is receiving care or services from VHA, or which resulted from treatment of that medical condition, e.g., stroke, poly trauma, traumatic brain injury, diabetes, multiple sclerosis, vascular disease, geriatric chronic illnesses, toxicity from drugs, ocular photosensitivity from drugs, cataract surgery, and/or other surgeries performed on the eye, ear, or brain resulting in vision or hearing impairment.

(g) Those with significant functional or cognitive impairment evidenced by deficiencies in the ability to perform activities of daily living.

(h) Those that have vision and/or hearing impairment severe enough that it interferes with their ability to participate actively in their own medical treatment and to reduce the impact of dual sensory impairment (combined hearing and vision loss).

Note: The term "severe" is to be interpreted as a vision and/or hearing loss that interferes with or restricts access to, involvement in, or active participation in health care services (e.g., communication or reading medication labels). The term is not to be interpreted to mean that a severe hearing or vision loss must exist to be eligible for hearing aids or eyeglasses. Those veterans who have service connected vision disabilities rated zero percent; or service connected hearing disabilities rated zero percent if there is organic conductive, mixed, or sensory hearing impairment, and loss of pure tone hearing sensitivity in the low, mid, or high frequency range or a combination of frequency ranges which contribute to a loss of communication ability; however, hearing aids are to be provided only as needed for the service connected hearing disability."

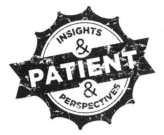

In part of the country where I practice ENT, there are two V.A. clinics in the area that have audiology and hearing aid dispensing services, but there is no local V.A. ENT physician to perform hearing evaluations. Because of the V.A. clinics issue, I often see veterans in my private clinic for complete ear examinations and hearing evaluations to determine whether or not they have hearing loss and to determine whether or not it is service connected. With the recent wars in Iraq and Afghanistan, I am seeing many more veterans in my office with hearing problems.

So, if you are thinking, "But I'm not a Veteran, what are **my** options?" Don't worry; there are other ways to obtain free hearing aids.

You may be able to obtain free hearing aids through your state's **Medicaid program** which may be run under the Affordable Care Act (Obamacare) provisions. This program is either a federal or jointly run federal/state need-based medical care program. The "benchmark plans" for each state covering hearing aids specify the minimum requirements for the qualified health plans that may be offered on the exchange in that state. The eligibility rules under the Affordable Care Act are different for each state, but most states offer coverage for adults with children at some income level. For adults and children, hearing aid services vary greatly between states and between qualified health plans.

Another option for obtaining hearing aids for free is through **your employer** (if you are exposed to industrial noise). Each year, I see dozens of patients who have hearing loss which is at least partially due to noise from their work environment. If your hearing loss is at least partially due to noise exposure while at work, you may be eligible for worker's compensation in the form of free hearing aids. Individuals who work in noisy environments like factory workers, heavy equipment operators, farmers, construction workers, law enforcement, as well as workers in many other noisy professions may qualify for hearing aids through worker's compensation insurance programs.

It is important to note that obtaining hearing aids through Medicaid-qualified health plans can be a complicated process. Each qualified health plan that participates has its own rules to qualify, as well as limits on how many hearing aids can be obtained. There are varying guidelines on how often they can be replaced, repaired, etc. Nevertheless, if you can locate a participating hearing aid provider in your qualified health plan, you have some patience and are willing to go through the evaluation process, it is a great way to hear better at little or no cost!

Most workplaces are compliant with OSHA laws requiring workers to wear hearing protection. Despite workplace noise abatement compliance, hearing loss can still occur. If you are exposed to 8 hours or more of sounds greater than 85 dB, noise protection is required in the form of ear plugs or ear muffs (or both). I sometimes see noise induced hearing loss despite consistent use of hearing protection due to underestimated sound intensity at the workplace or inadequate hearing protection. Most companies perform a hearing test at the time of initial employment (this is called a "baseline audiogram") and then regularly test employees' hearing on an annual basis or more frequently if required. The employer must have an employee medically evaluated by a physician if a "standard threshold shift" (STS) occurs. A STS is a significant change in an employee's hearing status compared to the previous hearing test in three specific frequencies. If this happens to you, your employer can re-test your hearing within 30 days and must inform you in writing within 21 days of the STS. If you find yourself in this situation, it is important that you make sure you see a board-certified ENT physician to review all of your hearing tests, examine your ears, and to make recommendations to protect your hearing. It is also important for you to have a final audiogram performed prior to leaving your job or retiring. If your hearing loss is determined to be caused by your employment, hearing aids may be required.

Industrial noise usually affects both ears, although it occasionally affects only one ear in certain circumstances. If it affects both ears, two hearing aids are required, as well as replacement hearing aids every 3-4 years for the rest of your life; since the hearing loss is usually permanent.

Things to consider when buying hearing aids.

Hearing aids can come with a confusing array of different features. Like the purchase of a car, the more features a hearing aid has the more it will cost. In general, custom hearing aids (ITE, CIC) are slightly more expensive than BTE or RITE, since they must be custom made for you and are typically smaller in size.

Some hearing aid options include:
- Type and sophistication of the microchip (how many channels and programs)
- Disposable versus rechargeable batteries

- Waterproof case
- A multitude of different colors from which to choose
- Multiple microphones versus one microphone
- Telecoil
- Bluetooth connectivity
- Volume control
- Automatic volume control
- Earwax blockage prevention
- Digital noise suppression
- Digital frequency shifting
- Digital sound directionality
- Tinnitus relief program
- Wireless communication between hearing aids
- Patient assist automatic programming
- Remote microphones (like a lapel microphone)
- Remote controls
- Wireless telephone adapters
- Wireless television adapters

...and many more options.

As of the publishing of this book, there are 23 states that offer hearing aids and related services through Medicaid programs-

- California
- Connecticut
- Colorado
- Delaware
- Hawaii
- Kentucky
- Louisiana
- Maine
- Maryland
- Massachusetts
- Minnesota
- Nevada

- New Hampshire
- New Jersey
- New Mexico
- New York
- North Carolina
- Oklahoma

- Oklahoma
- Oregon
- Rhode Island
- Tennessee
- Texas
- Wisconsin

If you don't qualify for one of the options outlined on the previous pages or do not wish to participate in them, and if you do not have any insurance coverage for hearing aids, then you are in the situation where you will be buying hearing aids out of your own pocket. I shy away from recommending buying used hearing aids unless they are professionally cleaned, professionally programmed, fit perfectly, and they come with a full factory warranty. I prefer to dispense new, custom-fit, custom-programmed, fully warranted hearing aids designed specifically for my patients, which will last them for many years to come.

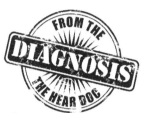

What are the basic features of a hearing aid?

This is what I recommend if you want to simply hear better and keep the costs down. First and most importantly, you need a **100% digital, fully programmable hearing aid.** This allows the hearing professional to program the aid for your personal needs. If your hearing changes, this kind of device can be easily reprogrammed.

Technology Differentiators: As far as technology goes, with almost every manufacturer, at each level of technology, regardless of the style of hearing aid desired (BTE, ITE, CIC, RITE), the price is about the same.

Style Differentiators: The style is based on your cosmetic preference, as well as on your type and severity of hearing loss. It is my opinion that two microphones are essential to improve your speech understanding and reduce background noise, unless a small hearing aid style (CIC) is selected which cannot accommodate two microphones.

As I have previously mentioned in this book, a **telecoil** is an inexpensive but very valuable option that I highly recommend. The only other basic function which I feel strongly you should have is a **digital noise suppression program** which will make your hearing aids much more comfortable to wear by reducing noise. **A warranty is essential with the purchase of any new hearing aid!** You should get a 2 year manufacturer's full warranty and at least one year of loss and accidental damage coverage.

In summary…when you buy hearing aids at minimum get these:

- 100% Fully Digital
- Two microphones (unless the smallest style---CIC--- is chosen)
- Digital Noise Suppression Program
- Warranty (including loss and damage)
- Telecoil

Regardless of which manufacturer you choose, they all have about the same functionality. As you move up into advanced technology (also known as "premium" technology) and add additional features, there are significant tweaks between manufacturer's products and thus the prices increase and devices can begin to dramatically differentiate.

Hearing aids can be purchased online, however, I do not currently recommend this. While an online hearing aid seller may look at a copy of your most recent audiogram to determine which hearing aids are best for you, an ear examination, hearing aid fitting, and personalized programming cannot be performed. Simply stated, once you buy hearing aids online you are on your own!

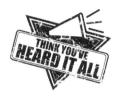

Consider Costco.

I love shopping at Costco. I am an "Executive Member" and spend at least $300-$400 each time I go there for office supplies and household items. I love the high-quality meats, fruits and vegetables I can purchase at a significant savings compared with my local supermarket. Did you know hearing aids can be purchased at a significant discount through Costco stores nationwide? It's true! Costco employs hearing aid dispensers and audiologists at about 500 different locations nationwide. Costco is now selling almost as many hearing aids as the V.A. system dispenses each year. One of the bright spots in hearing aid retail is Costco Wholesale Stores. Costco sells several different hearing aid brands at significantly discounted prices.

Costco Hearing Aid Centers offer quality hearing aid technology at a significant discount when compared to typical retail pricing through local hearing aid dispensers.

Costco employs both hearing aid dispensers and dispensing audiologists. Richard Chavez, one of Costco's senior vice presidents stated in July, 2013 that "[Costco is] now one of the largest, if not the largest, hearing aid distributors in the market." Costco has quadrupled the number of hearing centers in the past 10 years and now has almost 500 locations nationwide. As of this writing, Costco sells the following brands of hearing aids:

- Rexton
- Phonak
- Bernafon
- ReSound
- Private labeled "Kirkland" line.

They offer hearing aids with the state-of-the-art Bluetooth technology, as well as open fittings and traditional custom hearing aids.

So, you might be asking "How does Costco keep their prices so low?" It's really very simple; they purchase large (bulk) quantities of hearing aids from the manufacturers to obtain deep discounts. In addition, they hire a quality hearing aid dispensing staff which is paid a fair hourly wage. These folks don't make a commission, so there is no pressure to make you buy something. They also don't need to spend money advertising the product. According to Chavez they already "have a lot of traffic..." People already go to Costco for many other household products and enough customers stop by the hearing aid centers while they are there to make them a powerhouse.

Costco is frequently criticized by other local hearing aid providers; perhaps unjustly. Costco's line of hearing aid products is suitable for the overwhelming majority of people with hearing loss. That said, there are certain specialty products which are not offered, such as CROS hearing aids (contralateral routing of sound – for individuals with one hearing ear and one deaf ear). They are also criticized for not selling the latest and greatest hot new technology, but they do provide high-quality hearing aids with a full 90 day money back trial and full warranty.

In doing my research for this book, I also found Costco's Hearing Aid Center website to be excellent **www.costco.com/hearing-aid-center.html**. They have a wonderful FAQ (Frequently Asked Questions) page and many helpful instructional videos.

Overall, I feel that Costco is revolutionizing the hearing aid industry by providing reasonably priced, high-quality products which are dispensed by non-commissioned, professional staff. Because of this, Costco's hearing aid sales have grown 26 percent per year on average over the past four years.

Going with a Local Provider.

If you decide to visit a local hearing aid dispenser or audiologist to obtain hearing aids, I strongly suggest you review the following recommendations before you schedule an appointment.

1. Know who you are going to visit.

Do a little research before you leave home. Is the hearing aid provider a hearing aid dispenser, an audiologist or an ENT physician?

2. Know what you want from your new hearing aids before your appointment.

Be able to answer the following questions:

- Do you have trouble understanding your spouse or other family members/friends?
- Do you simply need help hearing the television?
- Do you need help with telephone conversations?
- Do you need hearing help in large groups such as religious services?
- Do you attend community meetings or business meetings with multiple speakers in a large room?
- What type of lifestyle do you have?
- Are you athletically active?

3. Bring a spouse or close friend with you to the visit.

Most hearing aid offices want you to bring someone else to the hearing aid consultation appointment. This should be a person whose voice is familiar to you and someone that is around you frequently. There are a couple of reasons why they want you to do this. The hearing professional may want you to try amplification with hearing aids while in the office and would like to see how well you can hear and understand your spouse/friend. Usually, it is the person's spouse that complains about hearing loss. Have a conversation with your spouse, the office staff, and even walk outside and try to have a conversation with traffic noise present.

It is also much more difficult for hearing professionals to "sell you" if a spouse or friend is not present. This is mainly because hearing aids are expensive. If you go to the consultation by yourself, you are much less likely to make a large purchase. Without a trusted advisor, chances are you will leave empty- handed. To increase the chance that you'll buy a hearing aid, dispensers have been known to sometimes offer free merchandise if you bring your spouse to the appointment.

4. Avoid the "hard sell."

Some hearing aid offices hire a professional "closer" (typically an outside salesperson). This person may or may not be a licensed hearing aid dispenser in your state. If possible, speak with the actual hearing aid dispenser/audiologist/ENT physician who will be providing your hearing care for the next several years to determine what type of hearing aid is best for you and what features you need to have for your specific situation.

A typical hearing aid consultation begins with a review of your hearing health history followed by a brief ear examination. Usually the next step is your audiogram testing. Once your hearing test has been completed you may be seated in a room with a "closer" who might use high pressure techniques to convince you to buy an expensive pair of hearing aids with more options than you actually need. Beware of this technique. Don't make the important decision about your hearing aids under pressure. It is OK to take your time and politely ask to speak to the local provider. If the salesperson stalls on that request or outright refuses, then simply get up and leave and schedule another appointment somewhere else. In many cases the outside salesperson (closer) will be promoted as a "factory trained specialist." Don't fall for the title. The person may indeed be trained at a hearing aid factory; however the techniques they learn to use to sell you hearing aids are perfected at the special hearing aid sales events. These events are typically heavily advertised, hosted by a local dispensing office and typically last between 2-5 days.

5. There are strict rules regarding hearing aid price advertising which vary from state to state.

For instance, in California, when a hearing aid advertisement states, "50% OFF" or "$1,000 OFF" the ad must also clearly state 50% or $1,000 OFF of *a specific price*. It must state:

- A specific amount or percentage off of the manufacturer's suggested retail price (MSRP)
- A specific amount or percentage off of the hearing aid dispenser's regular list price

If you see a hearing aid sales advertisement and the ad does not specifically state how much you will save off of a **specific** price, you should consider going elsewhere to purchase your hearing aids where the pricing is clear.

6. In most states there is no sales tax on hearing aids.

The state sales tax is usually paid to the manufacturer by the hearing aid dispenser when the hearing aids are purchased by the hearing professional. In California, this is definitely the case, but again this varies state to state. So, when you buy a new pair of hearing aids you are saving hundreds of dollars of sales tax. Also, hearing aids are considered medical prosthetic devices and may be a qualified medical expense for income tax purposes. In Washington, D.C., they have considered passing a hearing aid tax credit, but as of writing this book, there is no federal tax credit for hearing aid purchases.

7. In-home hearing aid sales are strictly regulated.

Again, the laws vary state by state. In California when hearing aids are purchased through a hearing professional in your home, there is a 3 day "cooling off" period during which you can cancel your sales contract and return the hearing aids with no questions asked. This is in part due to high pressure sales tactics which can be found in this industry. It is also safe to assume that most folks do not have a sound-proof booth in their homes to accurately test their hearing. Needless to say, unless you are housebound or have no other option, I recommend that you go to a reputable ENT, audiologist or hearing aid dispenser to purchase your hearing aids.

8. A FREE amplified telephone.

In California, there is a statewide program that provides a free amplified telephone (in both cordless and corded models) to individuals with documented hearing loss. The process involves filling out a simple form which needs to be completed by the hearing aid dispenser, audiologist or a physician. If you have a hearing aid consultation and decide, for whatever reason, not to get hearing aids, at least ask about this program and obtain a FREE amplified telephone. This program is offered in many states in addition to California.

9. Shop around to get the best price on hearing aids.

If a patient arrives at my office for a hearing aid consultation, having already had a consultation at another hearing professional's office, they are always welcomed. In many of these cases they want to know if we can match or beat the other office's prices. I always say, "Yes." Since we adopted a new (unbundled) pricing structure, our regular hearing aid prices are almost always lower than other hearing aid offices. Within the current retail environment the markup in most hearing aid dispensing offices nationwide certainly has room to adjust the price to make a sale. You simply must have the courage to ask! Typically you can save $200 - $500 per hearing aid. I assume that this is probably not possible at large retailers, but many smaller offices may be receptive. However, the only caveat is to make absolutely sure that you are comparing the price of the exact same make and model of hearing aid with the same features - "apples to apples" not "apples to oranges." It is sometimes very difficult to ensure an exact price to feature comparison because some hearing aids are sold with private labeling to avoid and deter consumers from comparison shopping. Another way to get a discounted price is to pay for your hearing aids with cash or check. Every retailer must pay credit card processing fees which usually vary between 1.5% and 4% of the purchase price. Ask the hearing professional if they offer a cash discount. With the current price tag for these devices any bit of savings counts!

10. Get a written purchase agreement.

A written or typed hearing aid purchase agreement should be provided with every hearing aid sale. At a minimum, this documentation should include the total price paid minus any discounts that were given, plus the price of any accessories or custom ear molds. If there is any insurance to be billed, this should be indicated as well. The trial period dates should also be clearly spelled out, including the length of the hearing aid trial (typically 30-45 days or longer) and conditions for return of the hearing aids for refund. This agreement should also spell out the warranty period and loss and damage coverage. If there is a deductible payment for loss and replacement of the hearing aids, make sure this is also spelled out, and that you understand the terms.

11. Check with your health insurance carrier and see if you have hearing aid benefits.

You may have health insurance with built-in hearing aid benefits. We have found that most health insurance plans do not offer coverage, however, a few of the higher-quality "gold" plans do have this benefit. Typically, unions and public employee health insurance plans have more generous benefits that may include hearing aid coverage. There tends to be about $500 - $1,000 per aid coverage, up to $2,000 total benefit--sometimes even more. Hearing aid insurance benefits often provide for replacement hearing aids every 3-4 years. If you don't know if you have this coverage, simply call the customer service number on the back of your insurance card and ask for the details of your plan or go to the plan's website (my staff has been known to do this for my patients). If you have an insurance based hearing aid benefit, you may have $1,000 or more that can be used to offset the overall expense of your hearing aids!

12. I've saved the best secret to buying a hearing aid for last! You can try new hearing aids FREE for up to 30-45 days in 30 states!

You read that right. There are currently laws in place that protect hearing aid consumers in all 50 U.S. states, and in 30 states there is a minimum a 30 day free trial period (in some states up to 45 days) - see **Appendix "50 State Specific Hearing Aid Trial Periods."** If after wearing the hearing aids during this allocated period you discern that they do not help you hear better, you are allowed to return the hearing aids for a refund. In California, where I practice, the law (Song-Beverly Act) requires a full refund of all hearing aid fees paid. In some states the dispenser may hold back a non-refundable "fitting fee," but that should be minimal compared with the overall costs. At that point, the dispenser is also allowed to try and adjust or replace the hearing aids to see if that helps you hear better, but in the end, if they don't genuinely help, you are entitled to a refund.

You can try brand new, custom fitted hearing aids for a minimum of 30 days risk-free in at least 30 states. Now, there is really no reason not to get help with your hearing and try some hearing aids. If you

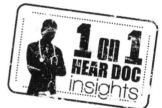

are fitted correctly, I believe that you will be amazed at what these tiny, modern devices can do for you and your life. The difference in your hearing may not be obvious overnight, but you have 30 or more days to decide if they work for you. In most cases therefore, <u>there is really no risk</u>.

Hearing aids always make squealing noises. They are uncomfortable, difficult to repair, and won't really help me hear any better.

FICTION

By following some simple maintenance measures, like keeping your hearing aids clean and dry, hearing aids will function well for years. If you experience a change in your hearing, digital hearing aids can simply be re-programmed for maximal hearing benefit.

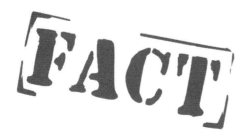

Chapter 13
Troubleshooting Your Hearing Aids

Challenges

Let's assume that you've decided to pursue better hearing, you've had a hearing test and a hearing aid consultation and you have now adjusted to your new hearing aids. Within days, you are hearing like never before. You love your new hearing aids and you are participating fully in life's activities. Your family and friends are happy and your spouse is thrilled. Then all of a sudden, your hearing aids start to "squeal" and create feedback noises. What do you do?

Hopefully, you followed my advice from earlier in this book and have purchased hearing aids with built-in digital feedback suppression. This functionality can automatically adjust your hearing aid's settings to reduce feedback noise. If not, there are several other things that you can do to make your hearing aids more comfortable to wear. Feedback noise usually results from amplified sounds escaping from the ear canal and getting back to the microphone to be re-amplified.

A simple way you can check to see if your hearing aids are working properly is to hold them in your hand. If you hear the feedback squealing noise, then rest assured that your hearing aid is working. Many hearing aid wearers check to make sure their hearing aids are working by simply placing their hand over their ear with the hearing aid in place, briefly listening for the normal feedback squeal.

Earwax

One of the most common causes of hearing aid feedback is earwax in the ear blocking the ear canal. Once the earwax is removed, the problem is usually resolved. Another common problem is a buildup of earwax in the hearing aid tubing. Removing earwax from the hearing aid is a simple process. Just use the removal/cleaning tool you received with your device or replace the removable earwax filter which is available with most company's products.

The battery and battery compartment on the device

Another common hearing aid problem that I see is broken or missing battery doors. The battery door is a tiny, plastic, moveable part and it must be opened gently with a fingernail or gentle pressure from your finger. In patients with manual dexterity problems, opening the battery door to replace a battery can be difficult and sometimes results in it accidentally getting broken off. I also frequently see patients who insert hearing aid batteries into the battery compartment upside down, which prevents proper closure of the battery door and often damages the battery contacts in the aid as well. If you inadvertently do this, avoid forcing the battery door closed as this will result in further damage. Remember that if the battery is installed properly, the battery door should easily snap shut and fit perfectly into place. If you must use more force or it keeps opening, it is likely that your battery has been put in the wrong way. If the door does break off or won't shut properly, your local hearing professional can easily repair it. Since this is a common problem, most dispensers keep a supply of replacement battery doors on hand to quickly remedy the problem.

The lack of waterproof casing

The hearing aid case can also be inadvertently broken or cracked. This is a much more serious problem than a broken battery door. Even if the device still functions properly, moisture can enter the cracked casing and slowly deteriorate the hearing aid's performance. With today's lightweight, comfortable, on-the-ear hearing aid designs, I have also seen many patients who simply forget that they are wearing them. Patients have inadvertently walked into a shower or jumped into a swimming pool with their hearing aids still in their ears! The result is water damage to the devices. Water-resistant hearing aids are now available; however the vast majority of hearing aids sold today are easily damaged by water and moisture exposure. I always tell new hearing aid wearers that the most important thing to remember about hearing aid maintenance is to **keep them dry**. I recommend leaving them out at night and opening the battery door to dry out any moisture which may have accumulated over the day. I also recommend a low cost hearing aid drying unit ($45-$125) which wicks moisture out of your hearing aid and can significantly extend the life of a hearing aid.

A poorly fit hearing aid

Hearing aids must have both a comfortable physical fit as well as a comfortable acoustic fit in order to be enjoyable to wear on a daily basis. With today's digital hearing aid programming, the sound amplification programs often result in a very comfortable and natural listening experience. That said, the physical fit of the hearing aid may still cause some problems. One of the reasons I often recommend on-the-ear hearing aids, with the receiver in the ear canal, is that they are very comfortable to wear. The hearing aid is usually connected to the ear canal by a soft, pliable silicone "dome" which is easily inserted. These domes are available in a wide variety of sizes to suit all types of ears. Custom hearing aids, which require an ear mold to manufacture, can sometimes be uncomfortable to wear. If a custom hearing aid or earmold rubs on a prominence of the outer ear or ear canal it can cause discomfort or a "hot spot". This is more of a problem in patients that have a hard outer ear (pinna) versus a soft, pliable outer ear. To help ensure a comfortable fit, when custom hearing aids or ear molds are ordered, the hearing professional must specify on the order form whether the patient's outer ears are soft, firm or hard. When a custom hearing aid has an uncomfortable fit or creates a "hot spot," the problem can often be resolved by modifying the earmold or hearing aid case with simple buffing by the hearing professional in the office.

If simple, in-office techniques do not result in a comfortable fit, you should insist on a "re-make" of the custom aid or earmold and a new ear impression. With custom ear impressions, it is important to ask your hearing professional if he/she would like you to close or open your mouth. The jaw joint (temporomandibular joint) protrudes into the front of the ear canal. When an ear impression is taken, this can affect the shape of the impression. An ear impression usually takes 5 minutes or less. An open mouth ear impression can result in less feedback than a closed mouth impression, but can also be uncomfortable when chewing.

Warranty issues

All new hearing aids come with a factory warranty, the length of which varies between one and three years at no additional charge. There is often a deductible fee for replacement of a hearing aid which is damaged or lost and usually you are covered only for a one-time replacement. Additional year(s) of warranty are available for purchase directly through the factory or with third-party providers through your hearing professional. The cost of one year of additional warranty coverage for a hearing aid varies from company to company but averages about $150 - $250 and is generally a good investment. The insurance will typically either cover loss and damage of the hearing aid *or* comprehensive loss, damage, and repair of the hearing aid. Hearing aid loss may also be covered on your homeowner's insurance policy. One reason why additional warranty and replacement coverage is valuable is because I have seen many occasions where family dogs have found hearing aids and ate them! Although the hearing aids may be retrievable a few hours later, they are usually chewed up, damaged and unusable. Hearing aids are tiny, expensive devices that are often as costly as jewelry and should be considered to be insured in a similar frame of mind, to prevent loss.

Battery problems

Excessive battery drain can also be a problem with hearing aids, although batteries typically last from seven to ten days. In hearing aids which are equipped with Bluetooth technology and with "power aids" for profound hearing losses, battery life may be reduced. Fortunately, power aids are usually much larger to accommodate a longer lasting, larger battery. Hearing aids can easily be checked for the amount of battery drain by your hearing professional. This can be adjusted by turning off certain functions that may not be required for better hearing and result in prolonging battery life. Hearing aids must sometimes be "re-made" at the factory if they have excessive battery drain to fix a defect in the initial manufacturing. Fortunately, hearing aid batteries are inexpensive and are easily purchased at most hearing professionals' offices and at many retail locations. Some hearing professionals offer free batteries with a hearing aid purchase for one to three years duration or have hearing aid battery purchase plans that provide free batteries after purchasing a certain number.

Here is a chart of various common problems and potential solutions to help you troubleshoot:

HEARING AID COMMON ISSUES

HEARING AID PROBLEM	SOLUTION
FEEDBACK NOISE	Dispenser to clean and check
	Dispenser to adjust feedback control
EXCESSIVE EARWAX	Have ears cleaned by ENT doctor
WATER/MOISTURE DAMAGE	Purchase electric hearing aid dryer
	Dispenser send to factory for service
BATTERY DOOR BROKEN	Dispenser to install new door
EXCESSIVE BATTERY DRAIN	Dispenser to adjust/send to factory
UNCOMFORTABLE EAR FIT	Dispenser to adjust or remake
UNCOMFORTABLE SOUND	Dispenser to re-program
NOT LOUD ENOUGH	Dispenser to re-program
	Take another hearing test
	Consider more powerful hearing aid

There are several common hearing aid problems which can occur, most of which are easily correctable by your local hearing professional. These problems include:

- feedback noise

- earwax problems

- water/moisture damage

- battery door problems

- excessive battery drain

- uncomfortable physical fit

- uncomfortable or inadequate sound quality

In a few cases the hearing aid or earmold must be sent back to the factory to be repaired or re-made. Hearing aid warranties are invaluable to protect you against hearing aids loss and damage and I feel that additional year(s) of purchased hearing aid warranty is probably a wise and good choice to protect your hearing investment.

The vast majority of hearing aid problems result from bad batteries or earwax problems. When I look at a hearing aid that is not working well, these are the first things I look for. Usually, I place a new battery in the hearing aid and clean any wax out of the sound channel or receiver of the device and clean the ear canals. In most cases the problem is resolved and my patient goes home with happy hearing. However, a typical patient's hearing can change significantly over one or two years, due to the effects of aging, genetic factors, medical conditions and noise exposure. One of the beauties of digital hearing aids is that they can easily be re-programmed for optimal sound as often as needed. A repeat hearing test is often required to determine the patient's new hearing thresholds and speech discrimination scores. This information is subsequently programmed into the hearing aid to create the new (and more comfortable) hearing aid settings for maximal speech comprehension.

....

"Seeing, **hearing**, and feeling are miracles."

-Walt Whitman

....

"I'll never be able to hear as good with hearing aids, as I used to hear when I was young."

FICTION

You have read this book, and now know the facts and some fiction about hearing loss and how to improve your hearing. You have much to gain and little to lose by getting your hearing evaluated and treated.

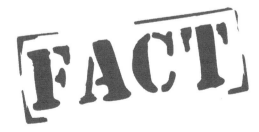

SECTION 4

The Beginning (Not the End)

Remember, only about a quarter of people who could benefit from hearing aids seek help. Even among hearing aid users, most have lived with hearing loss for over eight years before seeking hearing aids and by then, their impairment has often progressed to moderate-to-severe levels.

The following information is included in this section

- The future of hearing aids
- What do you have to lose?
- Better hearing leads to better health and happiness

In the future, hearing aids will be completely obsolete because the effectiveness of ear surgery will continue to improve.

FICTION

Hearing aids will always be a viable solution to improve hearing and they will continue to decrease in size and increase in effectiveness – and hopefully, prices will decrease to help more people hear well.

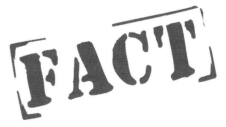

Chapter 14
The Future of Hearing Aids

So, what will hearing aids look like in the future? Hearing aids have already developed into amazing devices. Today's hearing aids are complex, tiny digital instruments. They quickly process and filter out unwanted sounds, automatically adjust volume, and amplify sound according to your individual hearing needs. All this sound processing occurs in small, stylish cases that come in a variety of designs and colors. These microchip containing marvels connect wirelessly to your cellular phone, TV, and other electronics and are powered by batteries measuring as little as 5.8 mm in diameter.

I think the hearing aid of the future will have even more sophisticated digital-circuitry, have a battery life of several weeks to a month and will even have capability to be charged from a remote device like a cell phone or remote control. I also believe that hearing aids will be increasingly linked to smartphones and other digital devices to seamlessly incorporate hearing amplification in daily activities for those that need it.

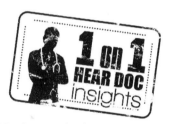

In the future, hearing healthcare providers like ENTs and audiologists will always be needed because of all the reasons mentioned in chapter seven. A complete hearing history and physical examination of the ears is necessary as a first step to restoring hearing. The ear canals must also be cleaned of any excessive earwax, which can interfere with testing and hearing aid fitting. And, of course, any medical conditions must be treated.

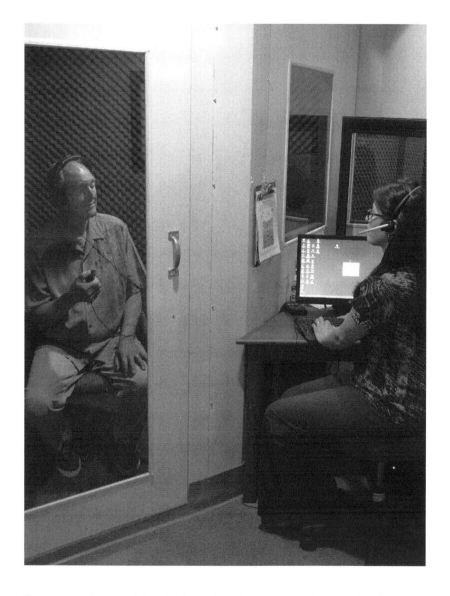

The testing in my office is done in a huge, sound controlled room (audio booth), but can also be done fairly accurately in a quiet room, without the audio booth.

The audiometer (hearing testing equipment) that is currently used in my office consists of high-tech audiology software which is run on a powerful PC. An interface unit connects the PC to the patient via the headphones or ear inserts. Unlike older analog audiometers which had to be regularly calibrated to maintain accuracy, the digital computer-based audiometers are 100% pitch perfect. Only the accessories (like the headphones) need to be calibrated from time to time.

Of course , there is currently no substitute for a complete diagnostic audiogram by a hearing professional. In the future, however, with increasingly accurate technological advances, I think this will change. Although self-testing is not suitable for all people with hearing loss, I believe that accurate, reproducible, internet-based self-administered hearing testing will become widely available. I believe that accurate self-administered hearing tests will eventually lead to better self-fit hearing aids, thereby reducing the cost of entry and opening the world of hearing to many more individuals.

I believe that computer-based hearing testing is already capable of fairly accurate self-hearing testing using internet based programs. There are several sites available today where you can perform a self-hearing test. Some of these sites include:

- **Myhearingtest.net**

- **Audiocheck.net**

- **Starkey.com**

- **Audioclinic.com.au**

There are also several iPhone apps that are designed to self-test your hearing. Here are some of those apps:

- Siemens Hearing Test
- Hearing Test Pro
- uHear

New apps are being created all the time, so do check for newer tests. Try using one of these sites/apps sometime. The hearing tests are very interesting and also very informative. The problem is that it is currently very difficult or impossible to ensure online hearing testing accuracy because of many uncontrolled variables like sound delivery system (headphones vs. speakers vs. ear buds), noise in the test environment, and lack of standardized volume controls.

Another major development in hearing aids is implantable hearing aids. These are not the cochlear implants I mentioned in chapter five. Implantable hearing aids, already approved by the FDA, are being used today on a limited basis. As of this writing there are two implantable devices available. One device is fully implanted and is called the Esteem. This device requires surgical implantation and removal of a portion of the incus bone. It is implanted under the skin behind the ear as well as in the middle ear. An outpatient surgical procedure is required for implantation and to replace the batteries. Another type of surgically implanted hearing aid is the bone anchored hearing aid. Bone anchored hearing aids have been available for many years. They are surgically implanted in the bone behind the ear and sound waves are conducted through the bone of the skull to the inner ear.

The requirements for obtaining surgically implanted hearing devices vary but usually include poor success with or refusal to wear traditional hearing aids. Of course, with surgically implanted hearing devices, there are the additional high costs of the surgery itself, as well as surgical risks like infection, bleeding, implant rejection, and anesthesia complications. Some health insurance companies currently do provide coverage for implantable hearing aids.

Another promising technology for the future of hearing loss treatment is stem cell therapy. This technique is not currently used in human trials. It uses embryonic or adult stem cells to reverse the underlying cause of sensorineural hearing loss; which is usually defective hair cells in the inner ear (cochlea). This process could conceivably reverse the underlying disease process and reduce or eliminate altogether the need for hearing aids. Inner ear stem cell therapy is still in its infancy. I believe that stem cell therapy may hold some promise in the future and could actually cure hearing loss for many in the future.

Sometimes people just need a nudge. In my ENT clinic, the audiologist and I help many people each month hear better by fitting new hearing aids. In addition, many more adults and children are able to hear better each month with surgical procedures that I perform. In writing this book, my goal is to help many more people with hearing loss. I hope that this book is simple, easy to read, and will help the reader understand why it is so important to treat hearing loss and how easy it is to treat (in most cases). Sometimes people just need a nudge to think about their hearing health.

Bill Clinton was the first "baby boomer" president of the United States. In 1997 as part of his annual physical examination, he had a hearing test and obtained two custom fitted hearing aids. Perhaps all his years of loud noise exposure, from concerts and band practice (he played the saxophone), finally caught up to him. I think it goes without saying, but obviously as president, it was very important for him to hear others clearly in order to make sound decisions with as much information as possible. When President Clinton got hearing aids, the rest of the US population with hearing loss took notice. The entire U.S. hearing aid industry, which had been seeing very slow annual growth up to that time, experienced a substantial increase in sales volume.

....

"Hear everything and judge for yourself."

-George Elliott

....

Even if I do have hearing loss, I do not need hearing aids, because most folks with hearing loss do just fine without any consequences.

FICTION

People who treat their hearing loss have major benefits, including improved interpersonal relationships, improved job performance, increased potential earnings, decreased risk of depression, improved memory, and an increased sense of control over their lives.

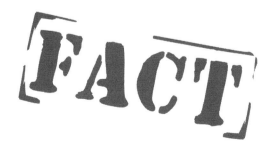

Chapter 15
Final Thoughts

If you remember only one fact, remember this:

Only about one-fourth of people who could benefit from a hearing aid seek intervention.

"Even among hearing aid users, most have lived with hearing loss for more than seven to eight years before seeking a hearing aid and, by then, their impairment had progressed to moderate-to-severe levels. Factors that influence whether a person chooses to wear a hearing aid include the perceived versus actual benefits, cost, stigma, and value (benefit relative to price) of hearing aids, as well as the person's accessibility to hearing health care..." – National Institute of Health

Have I convinced you that hearing is important yet?

I sure hope so. After all, saving your relationships/marriage should be at the top of your priority list because it's that important. But, there is even more good news: Getting hearing aids is not just good for relationships. Various studies clearly indicate that treating hearing loss with hearing aids can also improve:

- Earning power
- Safety
- Emotional stability
- Sense of control over life events
- Memory
- Perception of mental functioning
- Overall quality of life

Final thoughts

In writing this book, my purpose is not to convince you to buy hearing aids. Rather, my goal is to educate you about hearing loss and hearing aids and hopefully help you hear better by giving you the insight you need to ask intelligent questions if and when you decide to do something about your hearing loss. I argue that you have little to lose and much to gain by doing so. Remember, most people who do eventually get hearing aids wait an average of 7-8 years before doing so, and by that time they typically have developed pretty severe hearing loss.

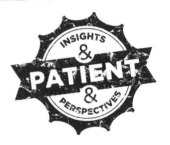

If medical or surgical treatment is recommended for your ears, make sure you understand the risks, benefits, and alternatives prior to consenting to any treatment. For instance, I occasionally see patients with ear bone fixation issues that result in hearing loss – who end up having a mixed hearing loss – that is a combination of conductive hearing loss from stiff ossicles in addition to a sensorineural hearing loss. The surgery will usually only improve the conductive hearing loss. Therefore, even if surgery to restore the conductive portion of the hearing loss is 100% successful, the patient will still have significant underlying sensorineural hearing loss which requires the use of hearing aids. In these cases, I usually do not recommend surgery, because hearing aids are risk-free and provide immediate restoration of both types of hearing loss, without the costs or risks of surgery.

Finally, here are the "Seven Secrets to Better Hearing"

Condensing all of the information, tips, advice and secrets in the previous fourteen chapters down to seven essential secrets/steps for better hearing-

1. **Know that good communication is essential to developing and maintaining every relationship.**

2. **If you think you have a hearing loss, be honest with yourself and admit it.**

3. **Take the first step and make an appointment to see an ENT physician or hearing professional to get help.**

4. **Treat your hearing loss with medical treatment or with hearing aids (which have the essential features I recommend).**

5. **Get hearing aids, for free, through the programs I mentioned or at reduced prices using the tips I provided and shop around.**

6. **Take advantage of the 30-45 day no-risk trial periods available in most states and receive a refund if you are not fully satisfied.**

7. **If you have normal hearing, and need help communicating with a spouse, family member or friend with hearing loss, use the active listening measures I have provided and encourage them to get help.**

If you are one of the fortunate few in the U.S. that have a local ENT physician, take the first step and make an appointment for a complete hearing evaluation that includes a physician's consultation and a complete audiogram by an audiologist or hearing aid dispenser. If hearing aids are recommended, you can wear them risk-free. Thirty U.S. states and the District of Columbia have between a 30-45 day hearing aid trial period, after which if you determine that the hearing aids do not help you hear better, they can be returned for a full refund (in most cases – see Appendix).

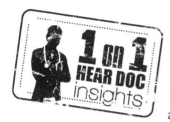

When you get new hearing aids, give yourself some time to adjust to hearing again. Take advantage of your state's mandated 30-45 day period to try hearing aids. Get used to wearing them, cleaning them, and replacing the batteries. Put them in every morning and wear them in as many different listening environments as possible. Wearing hearing aids is different than putting on a pair of eyeglasses. It takes time for your brain to learn to adjust to hearing again, especially if you have had hearing loss for many years without any amplification.

Remember to ask the tough questions of your hearing professional. Go back through this book and highlight parts that interest you or things that you don't understand. When you see a professional, ask questions and get some answers. I like it when patients come to see me prepared with a list of 4 or 5 specific questions about their ears or hearing. The questions tend to be easy for me (as an ENT physician) to answer and most patients leave the office with a much better understanding of how they hear and ways that will help them hear better.

In this book, I have answered the majority of questions that patients have asked me about hearing loss over the past 20 years. It is important to me to state again that most patients with hearing loss don't need ear surgery, but simply need to be fitted with hearing aids in order to start hearing better. If you decide to purchase hearing aids, don't blindly take out your credit card. Do what hearing professionals don't want you to do, but is in your best interest (with anything you purchase), shop around. Obtain a copy of your hearing test results and write down the exact make, model, and price of the hearing aids that are recommended by the professional so you can compare apples-to-apples.

As I have mentioned, the hearing aid industry makes price comparisons very difficult by using techniques, such as "private labeling" and refusal to publish prices or quote prices over the telephone. It will not be easy to find reasonably priced, reliable, affordable hearing aids, but it is possible. You must first navigate the confusing array of full page newspaper advertisements, colorful direct mail pieces and tempting offers like "50% OFF MSRP," "2-for-1 Hearing Aid Sales" and "Trade-In Specials." You are going to have a lot of resistance to price shopping, but in the end you will save money, potentially thousands of dollars, and most importantly, you will start hearing better. Let me leave you with this ear-popping statistic on this subject from a recent Consumer Reports survey:

40 percent of those who bargained got a price break on their hearing aid purchases!

One of the most satisfying things that I do as a physician is to help restore hearing. There is a video posting on YouTube which features a 29-year-old patient who is hearing for the first time after having hearing implants placed. It is a very moving experience to witness, and patients are forever grateful. Check out this link to see the Impact: **http://www.youtube.com/watch?v=LsOo3jzkhYA**

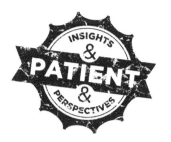

When patients with even mild hearing loss come to see me and improve their hearing through either surgery or hearing aids, they often improve their job performance, enhance their communication skills, increase their potential earnings, improve their personal relationships, decrease their risk of depression, have an increased sense of control over their lives, and generally have a better quality of life overall. It may take you years to recognize hearing loss, since for many, hearing loss comes on gradually. You then need to summon the courage to address your hearing loss.

I have personally helped thousands of adults and children improve their hearing using medical treatment and/or hearing aids. If you need hearing aids, forget the old fashioned notions about them. Today's hearing aids are sleek, stylish, powerful technological devices and when properly fit, they will allow you to experience life fully and improve your overall quality of life. By wearing hearing aids, you are telling your family and friends that you are too full of life to stop doing the things you love because of your hearing loss.

There are thousands of ENTs and other hearing professionals across the country ready to help you. There are over 40 million Americans who have some degree of hearing loss. For the vast majority, medical treatment or professionally fitted hearing aids offer amazing benefits.

Take the first step and schedule a hearing test and consultation with a local hearing professional. If you have a local ENT doctor, I personally think that's the best place to start. If not, look for an audiologist or a hearing aid dispenser. Whatever you do, don't put off restoring your hearing for several years like so many do. Even though this is the end of this book, it is just the beginning for you to achieve the full benefits of better hearing. Remember, hearing aids are exactly that, an aid to your hearing. No, they will not usually restore the hearing of your youth, but they are guaranteed in over 30 states and the District of Columbia to help you hear better than you are hearing now. Start living life to the fullest. Don't push your hearing down to the bottom of your priority list, next to getting your teeth cleaned. Take years off your physiological age by simply improving your hearing.

Thanks for listening and…

Happy Hearing!
Timothy Frantz, M.D.
"The Hear Doc™"

Appendices

Within Earshot (Tools to Use)

Better hearing is now within earshot. To make sure you have a consolidated place for reference of some of the items, terms and definitions mentioned throughout this book, I have created the following appendices. This will be a good place to help keep you motivated, inspired and educated on your continued journey to better hearing.

The following information is contained in the appendices:

- Testimonials and Stories
- Assessments
- Hearing Aid Trial Guidelines for all 50 States and D.C.
- Glossary

Stories and Testimonials

Here are some real life examples, from my practice, of how restoring hearing can improve your life:

Stories

Henry, a gentleman in his late-seventies, came in for a hearing evaluation with his grandson. It was apparent the two had a close relationship and Henry seemed content to let his grandson do most of the talking for him. The grandson expressed that he hoped hearing aids would provide his grandpa with a better quality of life. Apparently, Henry used to be the life of the party but was becoming more withdrawn due to his hearing loss. Two weeks later at his first follow-up, after being fitted with hearing aids, his grandson cracked a joke to which Henry immediately popped back a comment of his own. The bantering continued throughout the visit. At his next follow up appointment, Henry confidently came in on his own. The ability to hear better had provided Henry with more independence and the ability to interact with his family.

Testimonials

"Thank you so much for my new hearing aids. I knew for a couple of years that I needed to do something about my hearing, but I kept putting it off. Now I wish I hadn't, because it has been a joy hearing again. Helen's voice is much clearer to me now and we can actually have a conversation in a restaurant. The hearing aids make the soft sounds louder for me and make the loud background sounds softer. Thanks again."   -Fred L

"I have counted on Dr. Frantz for years to help with my hearing problems. He has always been so helpful to me, as I tend to ask a lot of questions. In every appointment I've ever had, Dr. Frantz explains things to me in a way that helps me really understand. I've been to a lot of doctors over the years and, by far, Dr. Frantz is the nicest of them all. He's so passionate about making sure that I hear better when I walk out his office door."
-Sharon M.

"For years I had to put up with my husband's poor hearing. I can't tell you how frustrating that was. I kept telling him that it was a problem for him, me, and our friends and family. Finally, I got him to visit with Dr. Frantz. It was instantly clear that Dr. Frantz has dealt with many people who have hearing loss, but are in denial. He was wonderful with my husband. While he was compassionate, he really was able to convince my husband that his quality of life would be so much better with some advanced hearing aids. Let me tell you, our marriage has never been better! Thanks so much Dr. Frantz!"
-Mary L.

"After battling hearing issues for a long time I finally decided to check out hearing aids. The first place I went to felt like a used car lot. It was just terrible. The sales guy just wanted to sell me hearing aids—any hearing aids. I walked out of that place and called Dr. Frantz's office. What a difference! Dr. Frantz and his staff were good to me. They helped me find the perfect solution for my unique hearing problem. And now I hear better than I have in 30 years."
-Charles A.

"All my life I have had a problem with my left ear. I've tried so many hearing aids, I can't even remember them all. A few years ago, I moved to northern California and had the opportunity to meet Dr. Frantz. He really helped me hear better. He was able to find a hearing aid that fit my ear just right. I've been a loyal patient of Dr. Frantz ever since. I don't know where I'd be today without his expertise and caring manner."
-Rose E.

Hearing Ability Assessment Questionnaire

This questionnaire asks some simple questions which help me to determine whether or not a patient has hearing loss. These ten questions help me determine the likelihood of hearing loss based on the number of positive responses:

Do you have difficulty understanding speech in a group?

Do you hear people speaking but not understand them?

Do you ask people to repeat themselves?

Do others raise their voices to help you hear them?

Do you have to turn the TV up louder than normal?

Do you concentrate so much to listen that you tire from it?

Do you ever avoid situations because of your hearing?

Do you have difficulty understanding conversations in the car?

Do you have difficulty understanding on the phone?

Do you hear some people's voices better than others?

If you answered "Yes" to two or more of these questions, there is a high likelihood that you suffer from hearing loss. If so, please consider seeing an ENT physician or hearing professional to get help with your hearing.

Active Listening Measures

1. Turn off the TV/radio if you need to have an important conversation.

2. Move to the same room if possible. Do not try to have conversations between floors of your home or from one room to the next. Have conversations in places where you can be close to the other person(s).

3. Move to a quiet room with the least amount of background noise.

4. Tell others that you have a hearing loss.

5. Try to face others who are speaking (ideally 3 to 4 feet apart). I often hear stories of a spouse who "will not listen" even though one spouse is watching TV in the family room and the other is in the kitchen noisily preparing food!

6. Watch each other's faces/lips. Make sure there is adequate lighting to do this. Visual cues are very important to a person with hearing loss and can help you understand what is being said. Take advantage of the lip reading skills that you may have naturally learned over the years without even knowing it!

7. If you do not understand something that is said, ask for it to be repeated.

8. Have important conversations when you are well-rested and attentive.

9. Ask for important information in writing.

10. If you have hearing aids, wear them! Studies show that almost half of hearing aids are not worn on a daily basis.

50 State Hearing Aid Trial Period Guidelines

There are currently laws in place that protect hearing aid consumers in all 50 U.S. states. In 30 states plus the District of Columbia, there is a minimum 30-day free trial period (in some states up to 45 days). Below are the trial periods and refund guidelines for each state. If after wearing the hearing aids during this allocated period you discern that they do not help you hear better, you are allowed to return the hearing aids to the dispenser for a refund.

State	Trial Period	Refund
AK	30 days (60 days if dispenser is not a physician or audiologist)	Refund of full purchase price less 10% and cost of ear molds.
AL	None required. Right to cancel matter of sales contract.	Dependent on terms of sales contract.
AR	None required	None required
AZ	None required	None required
CA	30 days	Full amount paid.
CO	30 days	Refund of full purchase price less cost of material and manufacturer's return fee.
CT	30 days	Refund of full purchase price, but cancellation fee up to 12%.

State	Trial Period	Refund
DC	30 days	Refund of full purchase price less amount up to 5% plus cost of ear mold.
DE	None required	None required
FL	30 days	Refund of full purchase price less up to 5% and cost of ear molds (up to $150 - $200).
GA	None required. Right to cancel matter of sales contract.	Dependent on terms of sales contract.
HI	None required	None required
IA	None required	None required
ID	30 days	Refund of full purchase price.
IL	30 days	Refund of full purchase price, but restocking fee.
IN	None required. Right to cancel matter of sales contract.	Dependent on terms of sales contract.
KS	None required. Right to cancel matter of sales contract.	Dependent on terms of sales contract.
KY	30 days	Refund of full purchase price less 10%.

State	Trial Period	Refund
LA	30 days	Amount withheld from purchase price dependent on terms of sales contract.
MA	30 days	Refund of full purchase price less 20%.
MD	30 days	Refund of full purchase price less 10-20%.
ME	30 days, but 60 days for medical reasons.	Refund of full purchase price less ear molds.
MI	None required. Right to cancel matter of sales contract.	Dependent on terms of sales contract.
MN	45 days	Refund of full purchase price less a fee of up to $250.
MO	None required.	Dependent on terms of sales contract.
MS	None required.	None required.
MT	30 days	Refund of full purchase price less "dispensing fee."
NC	None required.	None required.
ND	None required	None required.
NE	None required.	None required.
NH	30 days.	Refund of full purchase price less fitting fee.

State	Trial Period	Refund
NJ	None required.	None required.
NM	45 days	Refund of full purchase price less contractual fee.
NV	30 days.	Refund of full purchase price less fitting fee of $150 or 20%, whichever is less.
NY	45 days	Refund of full purchase price less amount up to 5%.
OH	30 days	Refund of full purchase price less amount for expenses as specified in sales contract.
OK	30 days	Refund of full purchase price less 10% or $150, whichever is less.
OR	30 days	Refund of full purchase price less 10% or $250, whichever is less.
PA	30 days	Refund of full purchase price less 10% or $150, whichever is less, excluding nonrefundable services.
RI	30 days that may be extended by agreement in sales contract.	Refund of full purchase price.

State	Trial Period	Refund
SC	None required.	None required.
SD	None required.	None required.
TN	30 days	Refund of full purchase price less reasonable expenses specified in sales contract.
TX	30 days	Refund of full purchase price less amount specified in sales contract.
UT	30 days	Refund of full purchase price less an amount up to 15% (Hearing Instrument Specialist) OR cost of returning hearing aid to manufacturer (Audiologist).
VA	30 days	Refund of full purchase price less reasonable cost of audiology testing.
VT	45 days	Refund of full purchase price less 5%, up to $50.
WA	3 days	Full refund.
	30 days	Refund of full purchase price less 15% or $150, whichever is less.

State	Trial Period	Refund
WI	30 days	Refund of full purchase price less cost of ear molds and professional services.
WV	30 days	Refund of full purchase price less amount up to $125 for fitting.
WY	None required.	None required.

Source:

http://www.hearingloss.org/sites/default/files/docs/Consumer_Protect

ion_Laws.pdf

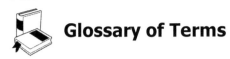 **Glossary of Terms**

Acoustic Nerve: transmits nerve impulses from the cochlea to the brain.

Acoustic Neuroma: a tumor of the acoustic nerve which creates hearing loss, vertigo and tinnitus and is usually not cancerous.

BTE: a type of hearing aid worn Behind-The-Ear.

Cerumen: also known as earwax.

Cholesteatoma: an abnormal growth of skin cells in the middle ear and mastoid.

Cochlea: the tiny inner ear, snail shell shaped structure which transforms mechanical sound energy into electrical nerve impulses.

Conductive Hearing Loss: a type of hearing loss which prevents sound wave energy from reaching the cochlea.

Custom hearing aid: a type of hearing aid which is worn in the ear which often requires an ear mold impression to be made for a proper fit.

Incus: the ossicle which connects the malleus bone to the stapes bone.

ITE: a type of hearing aid worn In-The-Ear.

Labyrinth: an inner ear system which controls balance also called the semi-circular canals.

Malleus: the ossicle which connects the tympanic membrane to the incus bone.

Microphone: the part of a hearing aid which picks up sound. One or two may be present on each hearing aid.

Mixed Hearing Loss: a type of hearing loss which has both conductive and sensorineural components.

Ossicles: the three tiny bones in the middle ear that conduct sound energy.

Ossiculoplasty: a procedure to replace or repair missing or damaged ossicles.

Receiver: the speaker of a hearing aid which produces audible sound.

RITE (or RIC): a type of hearing aid worn on or behind the ear which has the speaker in the ear canal also called Receiver-In-The-Ear.

Sensorineural Hearing Loss: a type of hearing loss in which sounds are not processed in the cochlea or not transmitted to the brain correctly through the acoustic nerve.

Stapes: the smallest of the ossicles which connects the incus to the cochlea.

Tinnitus: a sound heard in the ear(s) which is not present in a person's environment.

Tympanic Membrane: also known as the eardrum. It conducts sounds from the environment to the ossicles.

SELECTED BIBLIOGRAPHY

PREFACE

"Current News Releases." 15 Apr. 2014
http://www.hopkinsmedicine.org/news/media/releases/one_in_five_americans_has_hearing_loss.

SECTION 1
Chapter 1: The Importance of Hearing

Lee, Sarah H. "The Sound Of Mom's Voice Helps Kids Relax." The Huffington Post. 11 Jan. 2012. TheHuffingtonPost.com. 15 Apr. 2014
http://www.huffingtonpost.com/2012/01/11/sound-of-moms-voice_n_1200003.html

"Why is hearing important?" 15 Apr. 2014
http://www.oticon.com/hearing/facts/hearing/why-is-hearing-important.aspx

Kochkin, Sergei. "The Impact of Treated Hearing Loss on Quality of Life."
http://www.betterhearing.org/sites/default/files/quality_of_life.pdf

Chapter 2: Do You Have Hearing Loss?

Seliger, Susan. "Why Won't They Get Hearing Aids?" The New Old Age, Comments. 05 Apr. 2012.
http://newoldage.blogs.nytimes.com/2012/04/05/why-wont-they-get-hearing-aids/?_php=true&_type=blogs&_r=0

Chapter 3: How Do we Hear?

Silman S, Gelfand SA, Silverman CA. "Late-onset auditory deprivation: effects of monaural versus binaural hearing aids." J Acoust Soc Am. 1984 Nov; 76(5):1357-62.

Silman S, Silverman, CA, Emmer MB, Gelfand SA. "Effects of prolonged lack of amplification on speech-recognition performance: Preliminary findings." Journal of Rehabilitation Research and Development Vol. 30 No. 3, 1993. Pages 326—332.

Byl, Frederick. "Management of Sudden Sensorineural Hearing Loss." Otolaryngology -- Head and Neck Surgery May 1995 112: P150.

Chapter 4: Hearing Loss Prevention

"Noise and Hearing Conservation Technical Manual Chapter: Standards (App II:A)." Noise and Hearing Conservation Technical Manual Chapter: Standards (App II:A). 15 Apr. 2014
https://www.osha.gov/dts/osta/otm/noise/standards_mor e.html

Chapter 5: Ear Wax – It's Not Dirt!

Roeser RJ, Ballachanda BB. "Physiology, pathophysiology, and anthropology/epidemiology of human earcanal secretions" J Am Acad Audiol. 1997 Dec; 8(6):391-400.

FDA Consumer Update, "Don't Get Burned: Stay Away from Ear Candles." 18 Feb, 2010. 16 Apr. 2014.
http://www.fda.gov/ForConsumers/ConsumerUpdates/uc m200277.htm

SECTION 2
Chapter 6: Ringing in the Ears

Kochkin S, Tyler R, Born J. "The Prevalence of Tinnitus in the United States and the Self-Reported Efficacy of Various Treatments." Hearing Review, 2011, 18(12):10-26.

www.ata.org : Many valuable resources are available at this site and as a hearing professional I often refer patients with significant tinnitus to the ATA for further information.

Windmill IM, Freeman BA. "Demand for Audiology Services: 30 Year Projections and Impact on Academic Programs." Journal of the American Academy of Audiology. 2013, 24:407-416.

Chapter 7: The Importance of Seeing an ENT

"ENT-otolaryngologists." <u>US News</u>. U.S.News & World Report. 19 Apr. 2014
http://health.usnews.com/doctors/ent-otolaryngologists?sort=name&specialty=ent-otolaryngologists

"Consumer Reports magazine: July 2009." Hearing aids information, Consumer Reports Health. 15 Apr. 2014

http://www.consumerreports.org/cro/magazine-archive/july-2009/health/hearing-aids/overview/hearing-aids-ov.htm

Chapter 8: The Hearing Test

"Health Information Privacy." <u>Your Medical Records</u>. U.S. Department of Health and Human Services. 20 Apr. 2014
http://www.hhs.gov/ocr/privacy/hipaa/understanding/consumers/medicalrecords.html

SECTION 3
Chapter 10 : The Hearing Aid

Mills M. "Hearing Aids and the History of Electronics Miniaturization." IEEE Annals of the History of Computing 33.2 (2011): 24-44.

Howard A. "Hearing Aids: Smaller and Smarter." New York Times, November 26, 1998.

Levitt H. "Digital hearing aids: wheelbarrows to ear inserts." ASHA Leader 12, no. 17 (December 26, 2007): 28-30.

Hosford-Dunn H. "Hearing Aid Prices — Going Up? Going Down?" Hearing Economics. HealthMatters. 26 Feb. 2013. Hearing Economics. 20 Apr. 2014
http://hearinghealthmatters.org/hearingeconomics/2013/ hearing-aid-prices-going-up-going-down/

Chapter 11: Why Are Hearing Aids so Expensive?

Hosford-Dunn H. "Hearing Aid Prices — Going Up? Going Down?" Hearing Economics. HealthMatters. 26 Feb. 2013. Hearing Economics. 20 Apr. 2014
http://hearinghealthmatters.org/hearingeconomics/2013/ hearing-aid-prices-going-up-going-down/

Beck L. "Meeting Challenges of VA Audiology Care in the 21st Century"
http://www.myavaa.org/documents/JDVAC-2011- Presentations/Beck_JDVAC2011.pdf

"Hear Well in a Noisy World." Hearing aids information, Consumer Reports Health. Consumer Reports magazine: July 2009.
20 Apr. 2014
http://www.consumerreports.org/cro/magazine- archive/july-2009/health/hearing-aids/overview/hearing- aids-ov.htm

Belcher E., Freuler P. "New Avenues Break Cost Barrier." Hearing Loss Magazine. Sept/Oct 2013, pp 26-8.

Hughes, N. "Apple has sold 170M iPads to date, implying sales near 15M in Sept. quarter." 23 Oct. 2013. AppleInsider. 20 Apr. 2014
http://appleinsider.com/articles/13/10/23/apple-has-sold- 170m-ipads-to-date-implying-sales-near-15m-in-sept- quarter

Kirkwood, D. "Research firm analyzes market share, retail activity, and prospects of major hearing aid manufacturers." Hearing News. 3 July 2013. 20 Apr. 2014
http://hearinghealthmatters.org/hearingnewswatch/%202 013/research-firm-analyzes-market-share-retail-stores-prospects-of-major-hearing-aid-makers/

Chapter 12: The Secrets to Buying Hearing Aids

Hosford-Dunn H. "Regulation of Hearing Aids, part 4." Hearing Economics. 15 May, 2011, 22 Apr. 2014.
http://hearinghealthmatters.org/hearingeconomics/2011/r egulation-of-hearing-aids-part-4/

Klein C, Botuyan MV, Dyck, PJ. "Mutations in DNMT1 cause Hereditary Sensory Neuropathy with Dementia and Hearing Loss." Nature Genetics. June 2011. 43(6) pp 595-600.
http://www.ncbi.nlm.nih.gov/pmc/articles/PMC3102765/

"Prescribing Hearing Aids and Eyeglasses." Department of Veterans Affairs. VHA Directive 2008-070. Oct. 2008.
http://www.va.gov/vhapublications/ViewPublication.asp?p ub_ID=1789.

"Do I qualify for Medicaid, Eligible for Medicaid." HealthCare.gov. 20 Apr. 2014 **http://www.healthcare.gov/using-insurance/low-cost-care/medicaid/**

"Affordable Care Act | Hearing Loss Association of America." HLAA Updates. Aug. 2013. Hearing Loss Association of America. 20 Apr. 2014 **http://www.hearingloss.org/content/affordable-care-ac**

"General Information About Costco Hearing Aid Centers." Costco Hearing Aid Center. 20 Apr. 2014 **http://www.costco.com/hearing-aid-center.html**

Stock, K. "Why Costco Rules in Hearing Aids ... and Gummy Bears." Bloomberg Business Week. 11 July 2013. Bloomberg. 20 Apr. 2014 **http://www.businessweek.com/articles/2013-07-11/why-costco-rules-in-hearing-aids-dot-as-well-as-gummie-bears**

Chapter 13: Troubleshooting Your Hearing Aids

"Daily Care and Troubleshooting Tips for Hearing Aids." American Speech-Language-Hearing Association. Audiology Information Series, 2011. **http://www.asha.org/uploadedFiles/AIS-Hearing-Aids-Troubleshooting.pdf**

SECTION 4

Chapter 14: The Future of Hearing Aids

"Hearing Aids." NIH Research Portfolio Online Reporting Tools (RePORT). US Dept. of Health and Human Services. 29 Mar, 2013. **http://report.nih.gov/nihfactsheets/viewfactsheet.aspx?csid=95**

"Consumer Reports Insights: How to Hear Well in a Noisy World. "Washington Post, 23 Jun, 2009. **http://www.washingtonpost.com/wp-dyn/content/article/2009/06/22/AR20009062201623.html**

ABOUT THE AUTHOR

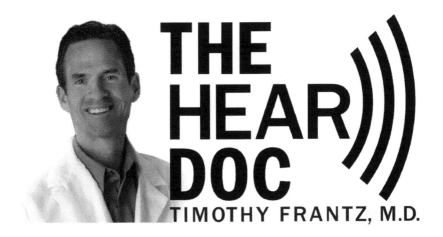

Timothy Frantz, M.D. – "The Hear Doc™"

Timothy D. Frantz, M.D. has provided Ear, Nose and Throat care to families in Northern California for over 20 years. As a board-certified Ear, Nose and Throat (ENT) physician and a licensed hearing aid dispenser, Dr. Frantz is dedicated to applying state-of-the-art techniques and hearing aid technologies in a caring and patient-centered environment.

Dr. Frantz received his bachelor's degree in biology at California State Polytechnic Institute, Pomona. He completed medical school at Rosalind Franklin University / The Chicago Medical School with high honors (Alpha Omega Alpha) as the senior medical school class president.

After finishing medical school, Dr. Frantz completed 2 years of general surgery training and 3 years of ENT specialty training in the San Francisco Bay Area with Dr. Raymond Hilsinger Jr. and his teaching staff. He served one year as the ENT chief resident. In August of 1994, Dr. Frantz opened a private practice in Red Bluff, California, and subsequently received his board certification in 1995. He actively practices ENT, dispenses hearing aids, and currently, has surgical staff privileges at several local hospitals. Dr. Frantz's residency research has been published in national medical journals. He has lectured both regionally and nationally on various topics. Dr. Frantz is a member of the American Board of Otolaryngology, the American Medical Writers Association and the Hearing Loss Association of America.

Dr. Frantz is passionate about educating and treating patients with hearing loss. In addition to this book, he writes a quarterly newsletter on hearing loss which is available at no charge through his website: **www.theheardoc.com**. He is available for speaking engagements, media appearances and private lectures.

Connect with The Hear Doc™

 The Hear Doc

 http://theheardoc.wordpress.com

 @theheardoc

Look for these upcoming book releases by Timothy Frantz, M.D. "The Hear Doc"™

"Childhood Ear Infections:
Does my Child Really Need Ear
Tubes? "

"The Hear Doc's Guide to
Buying Hearing Aids"

Notes

Notes

Notes

15903006R00129

Made in the USA
San Bernardino, CA
10 October 2014